PRAISE FOR

52 Life-Changing Lessons I Learned in Recovery

"These essays are tales of a spiritual unblocking; a colonic irrigation for the soul—something that may feel unpleasant at first before the true benefits unfold. In a world where we experience a constant feed of spiritual trends, the stigma of the word "god," and a default setting to be in control, these stories offer a calm oasis of spiritual simplicity. Lisa gives a master class in taking personal responsibility for our own suffering, illustrated by her own experiences, which resonate with me profoundly. This book is an irresistible invitation to open your mind, swallow the hard pill of rigorous honesty, and practice the liberating art of sweet surrender."

—Pearl, stand-up comedian, @rock_bottom_girl on Instagram

"Lisa's essays have a beautiful way of connecting to what we instinctively know to be true. She writes of universal truths, and so it's possible to open your mind and mull them over regardless of your spiritual beliefs in order to feel true alignment with yourself. Her lessons gently lead you from a place of victimhood, of believing that you are at the center of everything, to one of releasing the need to control and accepting accountability. It's really key in recovery to take a deep dive into all of these areas so that your sobriety is a happy and emotionally healthy one. So I absolutely love following Lisa's Instagram—all of her posts really make me think differently and deeply, and we could all do with more of that."

—Louisa Evans, therapist & host of *The Sober Rebel* Podcast, @stepping_into_sobriety on Instagram

"Highly engaging and personable, touching on questions I have always had but have never spoken out loud before. A thought-provoking must read for the believer, but even more so for the skeptic of God."

—Alison Bloomquist, host of the *Thank God Pod*, @alisonbloomquist on Instagram

"Reading this book felt like having a deep conversation with my best friend over a cup of fancy coffee—except this time, she's dishing out life-altering wisdom. Who knew enlightenment could be so entertaining? If you're ready to laugh, cry, and maybe even question your life choices, this spiritual journey is the one for you!"

—Brooklyn Sherrill, sober lifestyle influencer, @soberbrooklyn on TikTok

"Lisa's words are gracefully empowering to say the least. I found so much freedom in my heart to both forgive and take accountability for things in my life that I might have otherwise easily blamed and dismissed. If you want words that expand your mind, open your heart, and ground you into truth all at the same time, read this book."

—Jennie Juechter, MS Professional Counseling

"Dr. Lisa Stanton is an intellectual genius; she is a driven, competitive, always-striving-for-the-best woman...which, as she highlights in this book, is not always the easiest or even effective way to "align to the immutable laws and spiritual principles" by which this world is governed, thus creating a life of suffering and resistance. As a woman in recovery, I can deeply relate to Dr. Stanton's story—her struggles, her inner battle with intellect, and ultimately, how she hit bottom, which led her (and me, and a lot of us in recovery) to God and to a life of sober, serene, usefulness to others. The story behind this book and how Lisa came to write and ultimately publish it is nothing short of a

'God Shot' and a truly miraculous gift of recovery. I pray that the right humans are touched by her words, her story, and the way God is so evidently moving through her life and changing ours in the process. I feel honored to know you, Lisa, and to walk this sober journey heart-to-heart with you. May this book bless the masses."

—Kori Hagel, influencer, entrepreneur, and host of *The Kori Leigh Show*, @korileigh

"You will be changed by this book. Your own recovery will be enhanced. And you will want to tell others about this book, just like I wanted to tell you."

—Karen Casey, recomvery author emeritus and creator of the seminal *Each Day A New Beginning*

"Lisa Stanton's *52 Life-Changing Lessons I Learned in Recovery* so beautifully captures the journey from the pain, isolation, and desperation of her addiction to a meaningful, spiritually grounded life in recovery. Lisa describes in such vivid and relatable detail her journey from agnosticism to faith. Her vulnerability and honesty are both difficult to read at times and profoundly refreshing. For anyone who is struggling with finding their way to the spiritual path of life and recovery, and with finding a relationship with the God of their understanding that is both practical and relatable, this book is a must read.

—John Curtiss, president/CEO and founder of The Retreat treatment center in Wayzata, MN, www.theretreat.org

52

Life-Changing Lessons I Learned in Recovery

52
Life-Changing
Lessons I Learned
in Recovery

A Journey Towards Sobriety, Honesty, and Radical Forgiveness

by
LISA STANTON, PHD

BOOKS THAT SAVE LIVES

MIAMI

For permission requests, please contact the publisher at:
Mango Publishing Group
5966 South Dixie Highway, Suite 300
Miami, FL 33143
info@mango.bz

For special orders, quantity sales, course adoptions, and corporate sales, please email the publisher at sales@mango.bz. For trade and wholesale sales, please contact Ingram Publisher Services at customer.service@ingramcontent.com or +1.800.509.4887.

52 Life-Changing Lessons I Learned in Recovery: A Journey Towards Sobriety, Honesty, and Radical Forgiveness

Library of Congress Cataloging-in-Publication number: has been requested
ISBN: (p) 978-1-68481-705-4 (e) 978-1-68481-706-1
BISAC category code SEL006000, SELF-HELP / Substance Abuse & Addictions / Alcohol

This book is dedicated to my mother, Carol, who is both my most enthusiastic cheerleader and my original editor, and to my husband, Kevin, whose depth of faith and wisdom inspire me and thousands of others in recovery every day.

Without them, this book would not be possible.

"If it is peace you want, seek to change yourself, not other people.
It is easier to protect your feet with slippers
than to carpet the whole of the Earth."

—Anthony De Mello

Contents

Foreword

Lisa Stanton has written a walloping good book for all people in any recovery program. She so eloquently shares her own story of troubled alcoholism and drug addiction, a story of pain and struggle from childhood on until she eventually wandered into her first recovery meeting. As is true for so many, though, what she heard initially didn't grab her full attention; so she wandered off, only to return years later with a different mindset honed by a host of harrowing experiences that were carrying her dangerously close to a life from which she might not have escaped.

The different mindset was quite possibly due to a bit of maturity, the additional pain of continuing to use alcohol and drugs so recklessly, and the emptiness of a life that looked on paper like it had so much promise. Lisa had earned a PhD, and she had a great job. But peace of mind and satisfaction with herself, her friends, and her family were definitely lacking. Desperation had escalated; and hopelessness coupled with loss of direction was now coming to the fore.

Fortunately, the next time she gave recovery a whirl, she was ready to succumb to the beauty coupled with the necessary work that a life free of alcohol and drugs requires. And she has wholeheartedly walked a straight and narrow path ever since.

The benefit for us as readers is not only that Lisa stayed sober, but also that she began writing about her journey, what she was learning, and how she was able to use what she was learning. And that is what comprises this excellent book; her lessons become our lessons, too.

There isn't a thing that Lisa shares in this insightful book that doesn't serve us in much the same way that she was served by the lessons she learned.

Having the heart and the willingness to share with us all of what has helped her says so much about the woman Lisa has become in this span of a few years of her own sobriety. Although I have been on this journey for many decades now, I felt refreshed by her lessons, her excellent explanation of her journey, and probably most of all by her commitment to making a difference in the recovery lives of all of us who choose to open the pages of this thoughtful book.

Recovery is first and foremost about one drunk helping another. Lisa Stanton fulfills that commitment here in a most stellar way. You will be changed by this book. Your own recovery will be enhanced. And you will want to tell others about this book, just like I wanted to tell you.

Karen Casey
Author of *Each Day a New Beginning* and many more;
see www.womens-spirituality.com

Introduction

I am not God, nor am I one of the smartest or most important people here on Earth, even with a PhD. Nothing revolves around me. I didn't make the immutable laws of the universe nor of life here on Earth. But I have come to understand that there are immutable laws of life here on Earth, and that when I align my life with these laws or spiritual principles, my life becomes radically different, radically better, and radically easier. When I don't, I suffer. It's that simple.

Yet, understanding and believing in the existence of these spiritual principles was not easy. My intellectual pride seemed to get in the way at every turn. I was educated to believe certain things about the world, most of which turned out to not be true. My whole understanding of the world and my place in it has been dismantled and rebuilt one lesson at a time over the last several years. One lesson at a time, my experience of life changed for the better. These lessons are the content of this book.

I know today that I learned every lesson at the exact moment I was meant to learn it, yet my life would have included a lot less suffering had I learned these lessons sooner.

The purpose of this book is to help you learn these lessons sooner rather than later. This is a book of spiritual lessons. This book is not a religious text; I don't ask that you be of any particular religion to read it, nor even that you believe a Higher Power exists. I don't ask that you be in recovery from alcohol, drugs, or anything else, nor do I ask you to call yourself an alcoholic or addict unless that is your preference, even if you are in recovery. I don't even ask you to agree with me, especially not the first time you read this book. All I ask is that you read with an open mind. Many of the lessons outlined in this book took me months or years to understand. Some I understood first in my head and then in my heart, whereas others I understood in my heart, and then they slowly traveled to my head. Some I still only understand in my heart, but I am, nonetheless, going to try to articulate them here.

This book is not meant to be read once and then put down. It is meant to be mulled over, discussed, and well-loved. If the lessons contained in this book hit you the way they hit me, there might be some you don't understand at all until one day when they hit you like a ton of bricks. All I had to do for this to happen for me was keep an open mind.

Throughout this book, I use stories as examples, stories from my life and from the lives of friends and family who have decided to walk this path with me. Sometimes the names will be changed to respect the privacy of these individuals, but the stories are all true. My hope is that as you read the stories you might think to yourself, "That has happened to me," "I have felt like that," or perhaps, "These lessons apply to me, too."

The book is divided into four sections. The first section, "Accepting the God Thing," begins with a mini memoir of my own story of hitting rock bottom and coming to believe, followed by ten additional lessons on my journey from agnosticism to faith. This section comes first because the basis of my journey of accepting a spiritual way of living is first and foremost the existence of a Higher Power who I call God. The second section, "Spiritual Diagnostics," includes eighteen lessons on addiction, emotions, mental health diagnoses, and common therapeutic suggestions, not as I learned them in graduate school, but as I understand and experience them spiritually today. This section comes second because understanding the spiritual nature of my mental, emotional, and physical suffering was paramount to my accepting spiritual principles as the foundation of relief from suffering.

Section 3, "Debunking Self-Help and Trendy Spirituality," includes fourteen lessons that allowed me to finally give up the endless cycles of self-help and trends in spirituality and settle into a relationship with God. After accepting that spirituality was the foundation of relief from suffering, I found it was easy to get lost in self-help as well as in trendy and secular spirituality. My hope is that the lessons in this section save you from these same years-long red herrings I experienced on the path to Truth. The fourth and final section, "Radical Forgiveness," features nine lessons that dive into the importance and healing power of forgiveness both of self and others. Although there are many foundational spiritual principles, none has had a more profound impact on me than forgiveness. It has changed how I approach all my relationships, my community, and my role as a human. So, this book ends with lessons in forgiveness, which I hope will serve as the start of a long and fruitful journey of healing and faith for every reader.

Remember, every lesson is just a story. There is nothing you must do or believe. These are just fifty-two stories from my life and the resulting lessons that I learned.

I also want to add this caveat. I am always putting myself in a position to experience spiritual growth. I am constantly having new experiences during which new lessons are revealed to me. I am regularly unlearning things I believed were true, and, as such, there may be deeper truths than those presented here that I have not yet come across. Nonetheless, the lessons here have radically changed my life for the better, and, therefore, I believe they have the capacity to change your life, too.

Before I learned these lessons, I was a self-centered victim, sure that much of the world was wrong and sure that trauma not only causes permanent changes, but also that most things qualified as trauma. Today, I am a woman who is confident that all I have to do is examine myself, take accountability, and pray to God, and suddenly nothing in life, not even the worst things, have to cause suffering. Oh, and if the word God startles you, don't worry. I used to struggle with the word God, too. In fact, I used to struggle with the existence of God in general. More to come on that front.

For now, my hope for you is that if you finish this book having unlearned only one thing, it is the lie that other people can hurt you. The most beautiful reality I have come to experience is that all my suffering is my fault. Every drop of suffering is my fault, and by extension, yours is your fault. Oddly, this doesn't mean that others aren't wrong, nor that others aren't behaving in ways that are evil, or that the circumstances that surround you are your fault, but it does mean that your continued suffering is always—yes, *always*—caused by you.

See, I told you some truths might be hard to swallow. Please stay. Your life might just change for the better, even if none of your circumstances do. All it takes is a little open-mindedness, willingness, and perhaps some desperation. In the end, if you keep an open mind, I promise you, too, will think to yourself, "Wow, life might have been different had I learned these lessons sooner." Let's dive in.

PART I

Accepting the God Thing

Lesson 1

Stories Can Heal, and This Is Mine

When I hit rock bottom, I was twenty-nine years old, and on paper, my life looked like a success. Having finished my PhD in psychology the year before, I was a researcher at a well-known school of medicine. My expertise was in behavior change, and I had authored publications that appeared in prominent scientific journals. I had been the graduate student council chair of the health psychology division of the American Psychological Association and sat on its board. I had been a finalist for a prestigious National Science Foundation fellowship. Before that, I graduated near the top of my class from an East Coast university where I was a Division I athlete and served as the scholarship chair of my sorority. I was a certified yoga instructor; I volunteered regularly for various community groups. Although I was single at the time, I generally had long-term boyfriends, all of whom were successful athletes or entrepreneurs.

At the time that I hit rock bottom, I also blacked out almost every time I drank, which was nearly every day. I drank before I went out, I drank while I was out, I drank after I got home, and I drank when I wasn't going out. I was sweating through my sheets and often wetting my bed. I was chewing up my time-release ADHD medication. I frequently took my public speaking anxiety medication just to calm the intense pain of daily living. I was going on dates and sleeping with men to feel less alone and occasionally wetting their beds. None of my relationships in that time period had lasted very long, and I had strained relationships with most of my friends. In addition, I had been diagnosed with various mental health conditions throughout my life, from ADHD to eating disorders to depression to panic and anxiety disorders. I had also been diagnosed with various unexplained physiological conditions ranging from IBS (irritable bowel syndrome) and food intolerances to spinal compression as well as alopecia areata, which at its worst manifested as six large bald spots that covered nearly 30 percent of my head.

But let me back up. I was born in south central Pennsylvania to two highly educated, financially stable, loving, supportive parents, both of whom I rarely saw drinking any alcohol at all. My family originally included me, my parents, and my sister Lauren, who is two years older. When I was five years old, my parents amicably divorced. We children never witnessed any major fights, and they resolved all of the child custody and financial aspects of their divorce without even using an attorney, other than for those matters that required one by law. Although the divorce was amicable, it left me with a lot of confusion and unanswered questions. Instead of voicing my concerns, I just shut them inside and pretended everything was okay until I truly believed that it was. The only thing I remember from the day my parents told my older sister and me that they were separating is a buzzing sound in my head, a flood of emotions, and an internal shutdown.

I don't know if it was related, but I know that by preschool, my first mental health issues were becoming apparent. I had separation anxiety related to my mother, which manifested as dreams that she was going to die. I was also consumed by that fear when I wasn't in her presence. After the divorce, I spent nearly equal time at my mom's house and my dad's house. But the separation anxiety meant a lot of tears came up when I went to my dad's house. I felt badly behaving this way because I thought I was probably making my dad feel bad or making him believe that I loved him less than my mom, but I couldn't stop the obsessive thoughts and the outbursts they brought on. In short order, I also had a phobia of stickers and obsessive-compulsive disorder reactions to light switches and cracks in the sidewalk. The sticker phobia meant I could not be around stickers without feeling complete disgust and experiencing heart palpitations. If there was a "paid thank you" sticker from the grocery store on a milk carton or Gatorade bottle as was common in the early 90s, I couldn't drink it. If there was a sticker on a piece of fruit, I couldn't eat it. The light switch compulsion just slowed me down, as I had to complete a certain number of flicks or an intrusive voice told me that something terrible would happen and that it would be my fault. It was the same with the cracks in the sidewalk. In short, long before the drinking, drugs, anorexia, bulimia, binge eating disorder, anxiety disorders, ADHD, and panic disorder, things in my head were already coming unglued.

At the same time, as odd as it may sound, most of my life was pretty good. Both my parents remarried, so at least I stopped worrying about either of them being lonely. I had new siblings whom I got along with all right. I went to a good private school with a close-knit community. I did well in school. I played lots of sports for local teams. My dad often took my sister and me to a Christian church on Sundays; my mom occasionally took us to a Unitarian church. I remember being a little confused by the Bible stories and lessons, but I also chose to talk to God on my own quite a bit. Both parents took us on family vacations. I loved cats. I played outside a lot and spent a lot of time writing and journaling. I had some pretty extreme lows, but I was also pretty okay a lot of the time, and to my understanding, I was mostly quite pleasant to be around. Perhaps I was a little precocious, inquisitive, and competitive, but otherwise I was quite pleasant.

I always got along better with adults than children though, and for as long as I can remember, I had trouble making friends. I was always in my head. I am sure there were others in my elementary school who thought I was their friend, I just always felt different. By third grade, I had one close friend named Grace, but that is the only one I can really identify. By fifth grade, I had a second friend named John, whose parents were also divorced. Although he went to my school, we had bonded mostly over late night AOL Instant Messenger chats.

One February afternoon, my mother received a call about a murder-suicide. John's mom had shot and killed him and then turned the gun on herself. The only thing that I remember is that same buzzing sound in my head and the same feeling of shutdown that I had experienced at the time of my parents' separation.

With that, the little faith I had in humanity and in God started to slowly fade away. I didn't understand John's death nor his mother's. Around the same time, my stepdad's ex-wife died of alcohol-related liver failure and a family friend died of cancer. There had also been a series of break-ins at my dad's house. Although they were limited to the front mud room and the separated garage, they left me in fear, and every time I prayed to God for them to stop and they didn't, I was left feeling lost and alone.

I was eleven years old and confused. Although my relationship with God had always been tenuous, in the face of all the confusion around me, it was becoming nonexistent.

But I was starting middle school, and I had bigger things to worry about. Middle school changed my social status. I found myself in a group of friends for the first time in my life. I was invited to sleepovers. I was sitting at their lunch table, which meant I was important. I had friends to spend time with after school and friends on my sports teams. At the time, I attributed my rapidly advanced social standing to becoming pretty and dressing better. I am not sure if that was true, but whether it was or wasn't, that belief set me up for years of friendships that I believed depended on what I looked like on the outside. Clearly, my new friends had not led to changes to my internal state, and I still felt alone, different, and confused. On top of that, I was living in fear that my outer beauty would change, and then I would lose my friends. By the end of eighth grade, I had my first drink.

That first drink was twelve ounces of whiskey. I must have been too busy worrying about what other people thought about me to catch the part in health class when they tell students that twelve ounces of beer is equal to five ounces of wine and 1.5 ounces of hard liquor. I had gotten a call from a friend before a going-away party she was hosting for another friend of ours who was heading to boarding school that fall. She whispered, "We're drinking!" I asked "What? What does that mean?" She answered, "Just drink twelve ounces. Twelve ounces!" Click. She hung up.

I am sure they each drank a beer, but whiskey was all I could find. So, I carefully measured twelve ounces of whiskey and chugged it down during the one-mile drive to my friend's house. It was only a few minutes before I threw up everywhere. But, as with many people who go on to develop an intense affinity for alcohol, the memories of that day were not stored as bad ones. I had finally found the key to loosening up, to getting out of my head, to being in communion with others, and to not obsessing about what everyone thought of me.

Perhaps not surprisingly, I began drinking whenever I could. At first, that was not particularly often because alcohol was hard to get. I would buy water bottles full of vodka from the neighborhood alcohol guy who sold it to teens in suburban cul-de-sacs. I would steal what little was in my house and from my friends' houses whenever the opportunity presented itself. By sophomore year, I had alcohol stashed wherever I could. I began drinking in the bathroom during school and even before sports practice and games. I was constantly blacking out. I was once almost expelled from school for being so drunk that I could barely walk during a soccer game, not one I was attending as a spectator, but one in which I was the starting center midfielder.

Tenth grade was also the year that I developed my first eating disorder. I honestly do not really know how it began. During my freshman year of high school I had been dating a senior, the quarterback no less. He was better at lacrosse than football, though, and went to college out of state to play Division I lacrosse. There were rumors that he was cheating on me even before he left for college, rumors that I chose to ignore. I know I had the thought that he might like me better if I was skinnier, but I can't really say that's how the eating disorder started. What I do know is that at the end of my freshman year of high school, I weighed about 115 pounds, and by that winter, my weight dropped to as low as eighty-eight pounds. It may have been lower, but that's the lowest I remember seeing. I am 5'6" although I think was only about 5'3" at the time. Either way, eighty-eight pounds was medically underweight.

I was sent to therapists and nutritionists, and it seemed that their main goal was to restore my weight to a normal range. That happened, but nothing else changed. I didn't really want to recover, I just wanted to stop feeling so weird. That's the only way I could explain it. I do not even know if I could have identified the feelings inside me as pain or anger or the need for attention, I just wanted to feel better. Obsessions like eating disorders, alcohol, and drugs kept my brain occupied, and life felt more manageable, even as I fell more deeply into despair.

My first "intervention" took place as I was about to enter my junior year of high school. I don't remember much because that same buzzing sound from my parent's separation and John's death clouds the memory of it, but I know that my best friend made it clear that she was going to boarding school and that the main reason was that she wasn't going to stick around to watch me die. At the time, my drinking had escalated to regular blackouts. And although I had probably gained about twenty pounds, that only put me at 108 pounds, and I still thought that a celery, grapefruit, and protein powder smoothie was a reasonable breakfast. In other words, my habits made it difficult to be around me to say the least.

Despite my escalating drinking and the way that the obsession of the eating disorder never really left my mind, I graduated from high school with a 3.8 GPA. That fall, I was headed to a university in Virginia where I had earned a spot on a Division I cross-country and track team. My weight had restored to a medically normal level, but I was deep in the throes of bulimia, exercise bulimia, and binge eating disorder. In other words, I would binge and then vomit, use laxatives, or restrict my eating; or binge and try to exercise it off, mostly by running; or just binge and fall into despair about the weight gain. My body was suffering. As a result, in the fall semester of my first year in college, a stress fracture formed in my shin that ended up turning into a larger break. I don't say that I broke my leg, but that my leg broke, because it just kind of cracked from some combination of drinking, disordered eating, and extreme stress. By that spring, I had decided that running was not for me, and I joined a sorority where my drinking was initially deemed acceptable.

My nickname in college became "blackout Lisa." And yet, up to this point, alcoholism had not crossed my mind. It just wasn't something that was talked about in the circles in which I ran. I knew that I blacked out and woke up in places I didn't mean to. I knew I lost my phone and credit cards all the time. I knew my friends and my boyfriend were frustrated. But somehow, I just couldn't see it as a problem, and I always found an excuse for the latest blackout or a lie to cover the latest faux pas. I would seek therapy, blame the eating disorder, get a diagnosis for some new condition, or otherwise find fault outside myself.

My first alcohol-related hospital visit was not until my senior year of college. It was a Valentine's Day party, and upon arrival at the party, I had taken fourteen shots of tequila to celebrate the February 14th holiday. Only a few months later, my second intervention took place. My college friends were fed up, scared, and confused by my intensifying blackouts. Two of them asked me to brunch, and when we instead parked in a Starbucks parking lot, I quickly realized I was a part of an intervention. They took me to my first recovery meeting. We walked in, and all I could think of was how different I was from everyone else in the room. Those people were not like me. Luckily for me, my friends agreed with me. To this day, I'm not sure whether they just did not know what to say or whether they really thought I might not be an alcoholic, but either way, we all agreed I did not have to go to another meeting. Sobriety avoided.

That May, I graduated from college summa cum laude with a fully paid fellowship to begin a PhD program in psychology at a university in Minnesota. I moved to Minnesota that August and made a few friends. I was sure that now that I was out of college and halfway across the country, my drinking would sort itself out. It didn't. After one night out, although I don't remember what happened, I know that when I came to, I had fewer friends, and the ones that remained were concerned. Somehow, the thought of going to a recovery meeting came to mind, and that Sunday evening, I attended my second meeting. This time, the differences between me and the other people in the meeting had faded slightly, but I learned that recovery meant complete abstinence. No more drinking or drugs, no coke, no mushrooms, no molly, no LSD, not even marijuana. They said I shouldn't think of it in terms of forever and to just take it one day at a time, but I couldn't hear it that way. I heard forever. They gave me a newcomer's packet, a book, and some phone numbers. They did all the right things, but I wasn't ready.

So, I left that Sunday night meeting, book in hand, and didn't return until Thursday. The only thing is that the Sunday was in 2013 and the Thursday was in 2020, seven years later. During those seven years, I moved several times, and each time, something kept me from throwing out or giving away the book from that meeting. Those seven years were full of ups and downs and of trying on my own to find a solution to my drinking and mental health issues. But, with each passing year, I could see it was all getting worse instead of better. Those seven years included police interactions that led to warnings and rides home but never to arrests, one more hospital visit for alcohol poisoning, and a stay at the psych ward after a particularly rough night out. Today I do know that most people don't interact with the police at all while drinking, nor do the police drop them off at their local hospital to be placed in a concrete room which locks from the outside. But at the time, that did not seem too bad compared to what happened to some other people who I knew really needed help.

Nonetheless, those seven years saw me spiral into daily drinking, intensifying anxiety and depressive episodes, an ever-worsening eating disorder, and even more confusion. My drinking was out of control. The food binges were getting larger, and I was binging on food that was not mine, even stealing it from roommates and friends. I was throwing food away and then digging it out of the trash. I had also developed a plethora of physical conditions no doctor could explain, from IBS to alopecia areata. In addition to the physical diagnoses, my mental health diagnoses included generalized anxiety disorder, social anxiety disorder, separation anxiety disorder, obsessive-compulsive disorder, panic disorder, alexithymia, and ADHD, among others. I did not know why everything seemed to be spiraling out of control, but I knew that it was, so I tried to control the external behaviors to the best of my ability.

I tried the classic means of controlling my drinking and eating; I made various plans, rules, and promises, but nothing worked for more than a little while. Defeated, I sought relief from my internal suffering in any way I could. I dated stable men, and I dated men who drank like me. I tried reconnecting with old friends and making new friends. I became a certified yoga instructor, and then I decided the problem was that it was the wrong type of yoga. I tried breathwork, ice baths, and infrared saunas. I lay on therapeutic beds of nails and went to a few acupuncturists and herbalists. I tried volunteering more. I learned about crystals, metaphysics, human design, channeling, tarot cards, manifestation, and healing my inner child. I went to several different kinds of therapy. I took a class to become a psychic medium. I took large doses of psychedelics and then tried microdosing. I changed my diet to vegan and then to keto. I went on cleanses. I would find short respites during which I thought I had unlocked the answers to life. But the end of each period of respite left me feeling more lost, anxious, confused about myself, and increasingly confused about reality itself and the meaning of life. During those seven years, I also finished my PhD in psychology and began a research position at a well-known school of medicine in Chicago. All was not well inside, but on the outside, all was well.

Within a few short months, everything would finally crumble. My life in Chicago had been reduced to drinking boxed wine and going on dates. I was lonely, confused, in despair, and showing up at work less and less. By chance, my job then went remote, so I didn't lose it; but as a result, my drinking became nearly constant, I was in a perpetual state of anxiety, and I was afraid of what I might do if left alone much longer.

So, I packed up my car and drove west, back to Minnesota, to stay with a friend who was also an ex-boyfriend. To my consternation, within a short time, he told me I needed to do something about my drinking or leave his apartment. So naturally, I went on a several-day-long drinking and drug binge on Lake Minnetonka, a nearby lake resort area full of opportunity to blend in while drinking excessively during the summer. It was Memorial Day weekend 2020, and although I didn't know it at the time, that would be my last major binge.

I woke up that Tuesday morning, and something had shifted in me. My friend offered me some wine, and I said, "No," a decision that may be normal for other people given that it was eight o'clock in the morning on a Tuesday, but for me, this was extremely out of character.

After sweating and trembling for a few days on the couch back at my friend's apartment—classic detox symptoms—I called a college friend whose husband was sober and asked him what to do. He told me to go to a meeting. That was the Thursday meeting in 2020.

By that Sunday, I had a recovery mentor to walk me through a program of recovery. Although I began working the through the program, I stayed stuck in many of my old ideas and prejudices. My vast education in psychology and metaphysics had garnered me the delusional pride of knowing that there was no God in any traditional sense of the word, and I wanted no part in that nonsense. Many of the young people around me at that time, albeit not particularly happy ones, felt the same way.

I worked through that program of recovery in a partially open-minded, half-trying manner. When I got to any suggestion of prayer, I balked and said things like, "If there is a God, I don't need to pray because He can hear me when I tell my mentor." My first mentor even told me it was okay to resent some people and to not forgive certain people if what they had done was really bad, and so I decided it was okay to do the program this way. Luckily, these half-measures got me basically no results, and seven months into my self-determined, God-free program, I was suffering more than ever. I wasn't drinking, but I was having daily panic attacks, my eating disorder had intensified to daily self-induced binging and vomiting, I was still playing around with pharmaceutical dosing, certain strains of marijuana, and even the occasional bump of cocaine, and I was not happy, joyous, nor free. I had started saying foxhole prayers to "God" out of desperation. I had reached my true bottom, the pit of despair where I found willingness and open-mindedness.

On Christmas morning, after almost seven months of trying to do recovery my way, I attended a recovery meeting in the most unlikely part of town and walked into a room full of joyful, friendly people who were laughing and joking with one another. I didn't understand. Did these people not realize how serious this was? As it turns out, they did, and they had found a solution that gave them a whole lot more than abstinence from alcohol and drugs. It was through this group that I found faith, as well as a mentor who'd had a spiritual awakening and lived in spiritual principles. These people weren't perfect, nor did they pretend to be, but they understood that God is love and that God is forgiving, and they too were aimed at being unconditionally loving and forgiving. We cannot transmit something that we don't have, and God walked me right into the arms of a group where faith was alive, well, and ready to be transmitted.

I can't explain why I finally became open, but deep down, I know those foxhole prayers had something to do with it. On that Christmas morning, I was overwhelmed by what I was told was God's love coming through these humans, and I was ready to surrender. I began starting my day with a prayer called the Set Aside Prayer. "God please help me set aside everything I think I know about sobriety, life, and you, so that I may be open to a new experience." And, little by little, I started to become open.

I knew that I wanted the joy they had, but I still just wasn't sure about this whole God thing. I didn't want to be associated with Christianity. I thought Christians believed that God was a white man in the sky. And I was sure that God and religion were one and the same, and that religion was a human-made construction put in place to control people. I was prejudiced, though I didn't see it that way.

A friend of mine knew a Nigerian Catholic priest and set up a meeting for the two of us. I was going to ask him how he, a Black man, knew that God was a white man in the sky, and so I did. He started laughing uncontrollably. When he gathered himself, he told me that he will never be able to fully define and understand God, and that faith is supposed to be a mystery. In that moment, my internal walls started to come tumbling down, as did my religious prejudices and my God prejudices. Although there was still a ton of work to do, as well as questions to ask and walls to break down, I knew the journey into the mystery of faith was the answer, and so I began that journey.

The meeting I walked into that Christmas morning is held Monday through Friday at 6:30 a.m. and Sunday at 7 a.m. Despite claiming that I was not a morning person at the time, I didn't miss a single meeting for nine months, and I still attend that meeting three to four times per week. Seeing the joy and love in that group and knowing that it came from their faith helped me gain a better understanding of God and what it means to be sane. Love is sane, everything else is insanity. On January 4, 2021, I got on my knees in a church and officially turned my will and life over to the care of God. I don't know if being on my knees was necessary or if being in a church was necessary, but it is my story, and it did change something for me. I still pray on my knees almost every day, and my sobriety date is January 4, 2021.

I also got a new mentor from that meeting, and I did everything my new mentor asked of me. When he said to write, I wrote. When he said to pray, I prayed. I finally understood what he meant when he said that common sense becomes uncommon sense. Common sense says you'll feel better if you blame someone else. Uncommon sense said that the solution was not for me to blame others for anything that had ever happened to me, but to look inside myself. I started to see that every disturbance in my life, past and present, was because of something in me, and that the number one offender was resentment. I saw that resentments in the form of anger, judgment, and unforgiveness were the cause of most of my pain, and that God could take these from me if I asked. But I had to ask, and getting to that point was the hard part.

I had to understand that the pain was my fault. What happened in each situation may or may not have been on me, but the pain always was. For example, I had to see that my parents' divorce wasn't the problem, my resentment about it was the problem. That required me to realize that my confusion about the divorce had turned to resentment over time. I didn't think I was angry about the divorce, but I knew I was confused about it. I came to understand that all confusion, if left unresolved, turns to anger and resentment. My mentor told me to think of the last time I lost my keys. I started out confused, but in a short time, I was angry. I saw that the same was true of events of the past. The confusion about the divorce, John's death, the break-ins, having trouble making friends as a child, and many other happenings had turned to anger. The problem wasn't any given event, but my anger about it and my unforgiveness of those involved in it. The hard part was seeing that. Once I could see it, I turned to God, and using the prayers I was taught, asked him to save me from my anger and for help forgiving; and I saw for the first time that everyone I was angry at had been suffering from their own pain. My heart softened toward them, and lo and behold, I was in a lot less pain.

I began to wake up to a reality to which I had formerly been asleep. I saw that I had sought approval from people, and then resented them when I didn't get it. Moreover, I saw that what I thought was people-pleasing behavior was approval-seeking behavior. I wasn't trying to please them; I had been seeking their approval of me. I saw that I had pushed people to their limit, and then I resented them when they retaliated. These realizations, however, were not morbid because I could finally see that with God, not only was everything in my past forgivable, but it was also possible to be unconditionally forgiving of others. I could finally see that fear was just lack of faith, and that giving my fear to God eased my anxiety and stopped my panic attacks.

Most importantly, I experienced that when there was nothing left on my conscience to avoid, I didn't have the desire to drink; I had conscious contact with God, whom I had previously denied existed. That same God eased me through a process of making amends to everyone I could remember harming, even those amends that seemed like they would be impossible. Each time I thought there was no way for me to solve a problem, I was right, there was not, and more prayer, less me, more God, was always the solution.

The spiritual solution that changed my life is not religion, but it is also not science. Spirituality is not something you learn; it is something that you do. It involved unlearning everything I thought I knew to be true about life and about myself. I thought that more education and knowledge would solve my problems, but those pursuits only took me more deeply into self. Instead, the path to serenity required the willingness to admit that I was wrong about everything I thought I knew so that I could enter the mystery of faith, where all my problems could be solved. I finally found the real key to loosening up, to getting out of my head, to being in communion with others, and to stop obsessing about what everyone thought of me.

The biggest lie I ever believed was that contentment isn't simple. It truly is. It is not easy, but it is simple. Every day I turn my will and life over to the care of God in the morning. I say a quick prayer during breaks in the day or before important conversations. When I get caught up in a disturbance during the day, I pause to see how I was at fault and turn to God first, then make amends quickly if needed. I talk to my spiritual mentors weekly and consistently mentor five to ten women at no cost to them, not because someone told me that I must, but because I cannot imagine not sharing the gift that was given to me. I end my day by cleaning up any disturbances remaining on my conscience with God and thanking God for inspiration and direction.

As a result of living this way, I no longer suffer from an obsessive desire to drink. Most days my eating disorder does not cross my mind—I wish I could say it was 100 percent gone, but I know honesty is most important, and it gets better every day. I no longer take any prescription medications, nor do I suffer from any of my varying psychological diagnoses. Although I didn't go deeply into it here, my IBS was extremely severe, and I used to suffer from debilitating stomach pains and even hives, leading to many visits to the gastroenterologist, an endoscopy, and a diagnosis of severe IBS. As a result, I eliminated many foods from my diet, but doing so provided no relief. Today, I do not have any dietary restrictions, nor do I experience any stomach pain, nor do I break out in hives. My hair also now grows normally despite there being no cure for alopecia areata. I was told that if I straightened out spiritually, I would straighten out mentally and physically, and this has proved to be true beyond my wildest imagination.

My family has also come back together and has begun to dabble with faith in their own time and way. I have watched more tolerance and forgiveness develop, often in places I didn't even realize it was needed. I no longer work in a fancy academic or tech job. I guess I write books now, and that journey has shown me that I am worthy because I am a child of God, with or without a fancy job, and that my job isn't my identity. I started riding motorcycles five months after getting sober and now take multi-thousand-mile road trips. I have closer friends than I have ever had in my life, friends who were my bridesmaids in my wedding to a stable, humble, goofy, loving man I never would have met without recovery and without trusting God. Our relationship is based on our faith and love of God, and we are very involved in the recovery community in the Minnesota suburb where we live. He is also one of my greatest mentors and teachers.

Most importantly, for the first time in my life, I have ceased fighting anything or anyone, including myself. My soul is consistently at peace. This peace has remained despite the ever-present excitements and tragedies of life. All I do is stay close to God, and by the grace of God, I now get to live life on life's terms. I no longer fight reality. There was a time where I couldn't imagine my life without alcohol, drugs, and eating disorders, without anxiety and fear, without unexplained medical issues. And now I can't imagine my life without God, without prayer, and without a community of people of faith I never imagined I would end up a part of but that I now call home.

Although this is the end of this mini memoir, if you wish the dive into the awakening part of the story was deeper, you have come to the right place. The fifty-one remaining lessons fit like puzzle pieces into the holes in this memoir. As you read through them, you'll not only come to better understand my journey to a changed life but also begin to see a roadmap for your own journey. So, if there is one thing I am sure of, it is that if you take just a few of these lessons to heart, your life will change, and if you truly manage to live by them all, you won't even recognize yourself. And with that, let's continue the journey.

Lesson 2

God Is Not a White Man in the Sky

It was a sunny winter afternoon in March of 2021. Although I had been trying to get sober since June of 2020, I only had two months of sobriety. And there I was, sitting on a screened in porch with Father Jacob, a non-Diocesan Nigerian Catholic priest with forty-two years of sobriety.

I ended up on that porch because I was in a massive internal battle with God. When I got to recovery, I was told that God could be the God of my understanding. Out of pure rebellion, resentment, and intellectual pride, I had proceeded to conclude that I was smarter than all religions of humankind and created my own God. The caveat was that at the time, I had not studied most of these religions at their most basic and elementary levels, let alone the beliefs of those with spiritual maturity who practice any of them. If I had, I would have known that Christians don't believe God is a white man in the sky. But, alas, I was full of pride and prejudice, so I created my own God.

My God was not a God but a Goddess. The Bible used male pronouns, so I chose not to. My God was also unconditionally loving. My God was forgiving. My God had a sense of humor. My God was always with me. The list goes on. I did not know that, for the most part, I had simply created a more limited and differently gendered version of God as described in the gospels. I thought I was creative and unique.

That day I found myself on that porch because someone loved me enough to try to hint to me that I might be suffering from judgment against religion, evidenced by my need to create my own god, and I responded to them, "Okay, so you want me to believe that there's a white man in the sky like Christians do?" I thought that Christians truly believed that there was a white man floating in the sky somewhere. Maybe some kind of a Greek god-looking figure, not that he necessarily looked exactly like a man, but I was sure they thought he had white-man-like features, maybe even a long beard.

I found myself on that porch because the person who loved me enough to hint that I might be wrong about some things set me up with a meeting with Father Jacob so that I could ask him how he, a highly educated, sober, Black man, believed and prayed daily to a white man floating in the sky. So, I asked him. "Father Jacob, how do you, an intelligent, sober, Black man, believe that God is a white man in the sky?"

Jacob did not respond to me right away. Instead, he looked at me blankly and then started laughing, almost uncontrollably. When he gathered himself, he looked at me and said something along the lines of, "Lisa, Lisa, Lisa, I don't know what God is. I have no clue. No clue. I have faith. It's a mystery. That is why it's called the *mystery of faith*."

I was floored. I pressed him about whether this belief was unique to him or whether all Catholics believed this. He obviously did not want to speak for all Catholics, since that amounts to about 1.4 billion people, but he assured me that certainly the mature ones believed as he did. In fact, he said that I should run from any man heard claiming he knows exactly what God is, because no man knows.

I was shocked. I had been both prejudiced and wrong. I had a long talk with Father Jacob, during which I learned that so many of my beliefs about what Christians believe were wrong. Christians weren't crazy. I was crazy. Well, some of them might be. But some people of every religion are crazy. And certainly, many people who claim no religion are equally crazy. Needless to say, there is no white man zapping people with lightning. That is a totally biased misunderstanding of God and of Christianity, Catholic or otherwise.

The lesson here is not just that God is not a white man in the sky. The lesson here is that so many of my prejudices against God and against religion were false. Yet I didn't even ask questions. I sought the type of religious people who confirmed my prejudices rather than those who opened me up to new understanding. I entered religious settings looking for how I could confirm my belief that religious people are hypocrites, rather than lovingly realizing that most people are just there seeking faith, hope, and love. The lesson is to keep an open mind and ask questions, because when I honestly seek, I find exactly what I need.

Lesson 3

I Will Never Understand God

Let me start off by saying that I don't know exactly who or what God is, and anyone who tells you that they do know is mistaken. Even those who have had encounters with God still don't know the totality of God. We have only a tiny human understanding of something that is so epic, so vast, so omnipresent, and so omnipotent that we are not supposed to understand.

God is so creative that God created creativity. Sit with that one for a while.

So, if I don't know who or what God is, why write about God?

Well, my experience of coming to comprehend that I will never understand God is an important part of my faith. Scripture itself does not even tell me who or what God is. It gives me images and portrayals of God. It offers stories of God both in human flesh and not in human flesh. But that still doesn't actually explain who or what God is.

I have heard it explained this way. Scripture points us to God and toward God, but scripture is not God. We look at the stars, and we see tiny specks of light, but that is not actually what stars are. We have only a minute understanding of the universe that Earth is in, let alone the entire universe itself, all of which God created. Scripture is what we can understand about God using words, but it isn't God.

Here are a couple of stories that were told to me that might help clarify what I am saying. Imagine a Deaf person is standing with you, and that you are trying to describe your favorite song to them. You can use written words to evoke imagery that might help them feel the feelings that you feel when you listen to it. You might describe how other people respond to the music. But your description will never be the music itself.

In a way, we all are the deaf person from this story in our understanding of God. We are trying to describe God using the five senses that we have, but God exists outside the five senses.

Are there times when I have heard God's voice? Yes.

So, God is a voice? Well, no.

There are times when I feel the presence of God, and it feels like peace and like serenity.

So, God is peace and serenity? Well, no.

We humans fight about God a lot, when we are all fighting about something to which we cannot know the answer. We just have to have faith. We have to pray. We have to seek God in the silence of meditation. We have to form a relationship with God.

I came to believe that it was possible that God existed by listening to other people's stories, and I came to believe that there was a God who loved me by spending time with God. I came to better understand the voice, feeling, and character of God by spending time with God in silence. I came to trust God by putting pieces of my life into God's hands and observing that they all were used for good in the end, even when I didn't understand the path or what was happening in the moment.

The only thing I can be sure of is that God is something that I cannot learn; I have to experience God. Scripture has to be experienced. Understanding the historical context is a beautiful thing, but watching God light up scripture in the moment for me is a completely different experience. So, every time I try to put God in a box, I remember that God can do more than I could ever imagine.

God is more than I could ever imagine. God cares about me more than I could ever imagine. God never asked me to define God. God just asked me to have faith.

Lesson 4

God Is Real

I will start by saying that I do not believe it is possible for any human to know for sure that God is real, and also that I believe faith to be one of the greatest gifts. So, although I have no way of saying with 100 percent assurance that God is real, my experience has led me to a deep knowing that He is, indeed, real.

Let's begin by getting a few things out of the way. First, from here on in this book, I am often going to use male pronouns for God. I have no idea why I or anyone else uses male pronouns to describe God, but as I grew in faith, it went from feeling odd to feeling right. In other words, using the male pronouns instead of fighting them has been a gift from God, one of many mysteries of faith. I have accepted that not knowing why is okay because my faith didn't come by understanding the intricacies of the Bible or any other book, it came by experience. Second, I do not believe that there is a literal being floating around anywhere, nor do I have any real conception of what God actually is. God just is. And finally, just because I believe in God as described, it doesn't mean that I believe whatever you might believe about people who believe in God.

So, how do I know that God is real? The journey began in 2020 in the passenger seat of a Dodge Ram pickup truck on a road trip from Scottsdale, Arizona, to Minneapolis, Minnesota. I had been working on getting sober for almost eight months at the time, and it was not going well. I had a vague sense of the existence of a universal energy that was greater than myself, but only in the new age sense. As part of my recovery, I had written a moral inventory and turned it over to the universe, not to God, because I refused to be identified with people who believed in God.

As such, my life was not getting better. My mental health was not improving. I was not enjoying life more. I was not freer than before. I felt stuck and confused. I had flown to Arizona to meet up with someone I knew from recovery, and he was going to try to help me as we made our way back to Minneapolis.

We got in the truck to begin the road trip home. I had my moral inventory in my hand—which at the time actually consisted of a list of person after person whom I believed had wronged me, that is, people I resented.

He suggested something novel—that I pray for forgiveness for my anger toward them. I was confused. I have to pray for forgiveness? What did I do? Well, what I had done was hang onto resentment and unforgiveness for many years.

He told me to just try it, and out of desperation, I decided to do so. He added an important detail: "Try praying to God though, not the universe." I rolled my eyes but agreed I would try. I had tried praying to God before, and although my beliefs wavered back and forth, some miraculous experiences had produced a degree of willingness in me.

I shut my eyes and began praying. I was not praying for them; I was praying for forgiveness from God for my own wrong. And something crazy began to happen. As I prayed down the list, prayer after prayer, warmth and lightness came over me. When I looked at many of the names, I no longer felt the pangs of anger. I started weeping for the first time in a very long time. It was working. I was actually becoming free from my resentments. I was beginning to feel love instead of anger toward the people on the page.

I began to have a real sense that God might actually exist. I described the warm feeling to my friend, and he smiled. He explained that he gets the feeling, too, and that some people call that feeling "grace."

I was bewildered. This was grace. Amazing Grace. No wonder that song is so popular! Grace is wild!

Amazing Grace, not just that day, but again and again to this day. The grace of forgiveness is how I am sure God is real. Remember, no one asked me to swallow everything else about religion, and what I have and haven't swallowed is an essay for another day. But I would be remiss if I didn't share my experience in all its fullness—the beginning of my journey to knowing, as well as any human is able, that God is, indeed, real.

Lesson 5

Try Giving God a Call

I remember having some belief in God as a child. I also know that intellect eventually got in the way; by my mid-twenties, I really couldn't understand why anyone believed in God. I thought that most people who believed in God were, at best, wearing some form of rose-colored, delusion-clouded glasses. At worst, I was quite sure that they were using the Ten Commandments (or whatever commandments their religion prescribed) just to chastise others and get people to believe they were good.

What I could not see was the truth. Why would believing that the world was created by an omnipotent being improve my life? Why would knowing that there is a divine plan improve my life? Why would the belief that I am unconditionally loved by an invisible being improve my life? And, if God really loves me, why do bad things happen to me and to others?

I had all of these questions, along with the tendency to only look for evidence that supported my assertion that belief in God was not necessary for existence and certainly wasn't going to improve it. I looked for evidence that people who claimed to be religious were almost universally problematic. I seemed to seek out evidence that they were more judgmental and less intelligent than the average person. My aim was to be among the least judgmental and most intelligent people on the planet. Religion, therefore, made no sense for me.

In all fairness, all religion is created by humans and is, therefore, inherently flawed. All of them. *All* of them. One more time, all of them. What's more, all humans are flawed, both those who are religious and those who are not. But I didn't see flaws, I saw reasons for wholesale condemnation of religion, and, therefore, negative beliefs about the idea of a relationship with God.

Here is the kicker though. Some of the calmest, most pleasant, wisest, most beautiful people on the planet that I have met do not believe that religious rules or a code of morals has brought them peace. They believe that a loving relationship with God has brought them peace. Most of them do participate in some form of organized religion, but they do not believe that attendance at religious services or even a specific sermon or homily will bring them peace. They know it is their relationship with God that does that. However, they also know that their relationship with God is strengthened by learning from and being in community with others who are also trying to build a relationship with God, and that God often speaks through those individuals.

But let me back up about ten steps. When I came to the low point in my internal life in 2020, having run out of my own ideas about how to fix my life, God became my last hope. I was cornered. I had to develop a relationship with God, in whom I did not believe. Some people have a white light experience at their low point, and that begins their journey. My journey did not begin with a white light experience. In fact, my journey began with a Google Voice number. I was so resistant to the idea of praying, while simultaneously convinced that I needed a relationship with God, that I decided the only way I would feel comfortable was to just give God a call.

I was barely ready to use the word God and certainly not ready to pray on my knees, so I got a Google Voice number that I saved in my contacts as "God." I pledged to call and leave a voicemail at least once per day. That was how it began for me. I wasn't ready to pray, but I was willing to give God a call. From there, I got tired of listening to the phone ring and was soon willing to pray. Then I became willing to pray on my knees and to call whomever I was praying to God. It was months before I was willing to begin to see that religious people might actually be right about some things, and more months after that before I began to actually willingly choose to explore religion for myself. But no one was asking me to do that at the beginning. I just needed to start to be willing to believe God existed and to begin trying to make contact.

All that was being asked of me was to be willing to put one foot in front of the other. My belief in God and my relationship with God began from there. If I could go from barely being willing to call God on a Google Voice number to openly writing about my relationship with God for strangers, I promise you, no matter where you are with your belief, you can get where you're meant to go in your relationship with God with just a little willingness.

For the record, all my fears that believing in God would make me dumber and more judgmental turned out to be false. I am actually less judgmental and wiser than I ever could have been without God's help. So, if you're struggling with belief, just try giving God a call and let it all unfold from there.

Lesson 6

Prayer Can Come before Belief

It was a cool mid-October day. I was on my knees beside my bed, as I assumed I needed to be for the best possible chance to be heard by a God I didn't believe in. I looked around to make sure that no one was watching, even though I lived alone. I began, "I don't know if you exist, but if you do, when someone is dying of cancer, I guess that is a pretty logical time to pray. So, I pray for your will for Judy. I pray that whatever happens, she and her family are at peace. If there is anything I can do to be useful, please just let me know. Okay, God, I think that's it."

It wasn't anything miraculous. I had been taught by my mentors at the time to pray for God's will for myself and others, something I still do today. I did slide in that little request for peace, but she was dying, and it was my first prayer in years. I couldn't even remember the last time I'd prayed with sincerity before that day, and I certainly hadn't prayed in the previous decade.

I looked around and got up. Not much had changed. Maybe I felt a little lighter. I wasn't completely sure. For the next month, I prayed a similar prayer every day. I wasn't ready to turn my whole life over to God, but I was willing to let Him take over this tiny painful piece of my life. Judy was the mother of an ex-long-term boyfriend, Dylan. She'd had cancer for several years, but it had escalated quickly. We were making juices and healthy meals for her and bringing them over to the hospital in lieu of the hospital food. We were Googling herbal teas and supplements. We were diffusing essential oils. We were open to doing anything that we thought might make even a small difference in her comfort. So, why not pray?

Although I was not thinking of it as related to my prayer, something strange began to happen over the next few weeks. I started seeing the number 417 everywhere. I would see it on the clock. I would see it on license plates. I would see it on signs. I would see it on menus. Every store seemed to suddenly have an item that cost $4.17. I set a ten-minute meditation timer, and then when I happened to open my eyes, the display showed that 4 minutes and 17 seconds remained. Each and every time, I told myself I was just creating this reality. I told myself it was just like that phenomenon of selective perception with cars. There are always red cars, but after someone shops for a red car, they see more of them. That phenomenon is real, but I was soon to learn this was something different.

On November 18th, I was lying in a tanning bed listening to one of my favorite podcasts at the time. A woman in Los Angeles was the interviewer, and she occasionally did solo episodes. I was listening to one of those. She had a lucky number that seemed to show up everywhere for her: 201. In this particular episode, she was explaining this to new listeners, and then she said, "But recently, I have been seeing 417 everywhere." I was so shocked that I sat up and hit my head on the tanning bed. This wasn't me just seeing things. I hit rewind and listened again. I'd heard it right, she'd said 417.

I had to tell someone now. My first call was to Christian, a close friend in recovery, who would be open to hearing about this miraculous sign or potential insanity of mine and would help me try to unpack it. I explained the 417 situation, and right away he said, "What do you need to accept?" I asked, "How is that related?" He told me to open the main text of the recovery program we were in. As it turns out, there is a well-known reading on acceptance on page 417 of the book. Interesting. I wasn't sure what I needed to accept, but I could perhaps figure that out. My daily prayers were not top of mind at that moment.

My next call was to Dylan. "I know you're super busy with your mom, but I have to tell you about this thing going on. It's just been wild." I explained the 417 situation and the acceptance reading and asked him if he had any ideas. He remained silent for a minute and then said, "Lis, I am not sure, but what I do know is that 417 is my mom's hospital room number." I couldn't speak. I had full body chills. Could God have been listening to my prayers? Could God have been using 417 to show me that He was listening? It certainly seemed like it. Moreover, I would soon learn that I needed to accept the inevitable end that was coming, but I would do so with the peace of knowing that God had this all under control.

Judy was sent home from the hospital that day. One day later, November 19th, she passed away peacefully in the presence of her family. *My prayers were answered, and I received my first lesson in prayer.*

God always answers prayers, just not necessarily when I want them answered or in the way that I might expect them to be answered. I thought maybe a miraculous healing would occur or that peace would rain down from the heavens. I didn't expect God to use 417 to show me that my prayers were being heard and answered. I had prayed for peace for her and her family; I had prayed for God to show me if there was anything I could do to be useful. Now here I was, telling Dylan and his family about 417, leaving them with the peace of knowing that Judy was well taken care of. There was no miraculous healing, but there was certainly a miracle of answered prayer around her passing.

The experience of knowing that my prayer had been answered was not only something I needed for me to begin to break the icy shell of doubt I had about the existence of God, but also, it showed me how the smallest acts of faith make me useful to God and those around me in ways that I could never plan or create myself. Telling that story to Dylan and his family brought them peace throughout their grieving process. Telling that story in recovery meetings has reassured others with similar experiences that they aren't crazy, and that God does work in mysterious ways. I have told that story from the podium at larger recovery meetings a few times, and the room goes silent. Although most prayers don't come with numerical signs, God knew that's what I needed in this case. My only hope is that allowing this story to live on paper gives you whatever experience with God you need today.

Lesson 7

The Problem with Church and Recovery Meetings

Now, before anyone loses their mind, I go to church on average about three times per week, and I go to recovery meetings almost every day. This essay is not meant to discourage anyone from attending either of these gatherings. Instead, the chapter title above is meant to convey an insight that is *not* about church nor about recovery meetings but instead about how people make use of them.

Recently, I was having tea and cookies with a new friend. I met her at a church, so it is perhaps not surprising that a major topic of conversation was our experiences with faith. In particular, our conversation was about how we each came to believe in God, but more than that, it was about the times when we'd decided to truly follow God's will and let God be a part of our daily lives and our daily decisions.

This friend had never strayed far from the church. She grew up going to church weekly with her family and had even continued to do so in college. She came to a point, however, when she didn't feel like she was getting that much out of it. She was going every week, but she couldn't figure out what the problem was. She wasn't experiencing the fruits of the spirit, like joy, peace, and self-control. Her heart wasn't changing. Her life didn't look like the life of someone who is in relationship with God.

I see this in recovery meetings, too. People go to meeting after meeting, sometimes more than once a day, but the people don't change. Some of them even stop drinking, but there is no change of personality. There is no rearranging of their beliefs about life. There is no innate altruism that develops.

What these two experiences have in common is that it can be really easy to show up to places where people are putting in work to build a relationship with God and *yet still not build a relationship with God*. You can show up to a place where the pastor is sharing about how to form a relationship with God, where hundreds of people are praying and worshiping God, and still not be forming a relationship with God yourself. You can listen to shares in a recovery meeting about prayer, meditation, and building a relationship with God and still not be doing any of these things.

Of course, there are churches (or other places of worship) and recovery meetings where people are not focused on forming a relationship with God but are instead focused on morality, trying to keep people from sinning, or trying to force others to change their behavior with fear tactics. Clearly, doing that is not bringing people into a relationship with God, but this essay isn't about those places, it is about sitting in a place where people are building relationships with God and expecting that by occupying a seat there, you, too, are building a relationship with God.

If that's you, let me be clear, sitting in that room will not lead to a relationship with God by osmosis.

If you are lucky enough to live in a country with religious freedom in churches or where recovery meetings are available, *the gift that you have been given is a chair and chance.* But nothing else happens just by your occupying that seat.

Showing up to these places and not actually building a relationship with God is similar to the following situation. Imagine that you've broken your arm pretty badly. You heard that emergency rooms are where people go to get broken arms fixed, so you go to the emergency room. You get there and check in. You even give your name and tell them you have a broken arm. You watch people go in and out. They get stitched up; they have their broken limbs set. But you don't actually try the treatment. You don't do the work. You just sit there. You come back day after day and week after week, and you can't figure out why your arm never gets better. Maybe you even make friends with the doctors, the staff, and other patients, and that feels good. But your arm will never get better if you don't actually do the treatment. Making friends at church and in recovery meetings is good, but it isn't a relationship with a transformational God.

Going to church or a recovery meeting without doing the work is a lot like sitting in the emergency room without accepting medical treatment. In order to recover, I had to accept the treatment, and it turned out that the treatment was not the paperwork of some specific program, the treatment was a spiritual awakening. I had to find a mentor to show me how to form a relationship with God. I had to pray daily. I had to look at my life honestly and confess my missteps to God daily. I had to share my faith with others. I had to talk to God and ask for His care and direction. When I just sat in buildings where people do these things, nothing changed, but when I did these things myself, my life changed faster than I could have ever imagined because I was finally in a relationship with a loving, transformational God.

Lesson 8

The Difference between Belief and Faith

As I began seeking a lasting solution for the existential confusion and pain in my life, I kept hearing about "coming to believe." There is no shortage of coming to believe testimonies at churches across the country and on the internet. And yes, I do know that coming to believe is a necessary prerequisite to faith; I can't have faith in something that I don't believe exists. But my life didn't change when I came to believe, my life changed when I began the journey of faith.

I came to believe at twenty-nine years old. Growing up, my dad had taken us to Christian church regularly. My mom occasionally took us to Unitarian church. Both families had Jewish roots. Although my relationship with God had been on-again, off-again while I was growing up, by my late teens, it had become nonexistent except for a trip to Israel in my early twenties, which was more socializing than exploration of God. At twenty-nine years old, after years of excessive alcohol and drug use, eating disorders, anxiety conditions, and bouts of general misery, I finally surrendered to the possibility of God. The moment I fully surrendered, a warmth came over me, and I knew I was home. But to be honest, it didn't really stick. For some time, even after coming to believe that God might just exist, and even after becoming quite sure this was the case, I didn't feel like it was working for me all that well. I wasn't at peace all of the time, or even most of the time.

So, what was my problem? *I had come to believe, but I was not living in faith.* Someone once used this metaphor to explain the difference to me. Let's say that I am brand-new to Earth and hungry. Someone tells me that grocery stores are how people get fed, how their hunger gets relieved. At first, I might be skeptical: "I have never even seen this thing. Could this really be the answer?" It sounds too unbelievable. I am unwilling to try it, and I stay hungry. But over time, I meet many people who tell me that they use grocery stores. Through their stories, I come to believe that grocery stores do exist and that they feed people. I finally believe!

Would I actually be any less hungry? Clearly, no. I must actually go buy food and eat it, not just believe it exists. At first, I might choose the packaged snacks or the hot bar. Easy, set prayers. Over time, I explore the produce and maybe someday try the rogue vegetables that the cashier doesn't even know the produce code for. In other words, I start simple, and over time, I develop my relationship with God.

Coming to believe is not how I made the shift from temporary peace of mind to lasting peace of soul. Faith is and continues to be how that happened.

I had to try, first in small, easy ways, to turn my will and life over to God. For me, this began with short prayers in the morning, at night, and throughout the day when I remembered. Simply just, "Thy will be done," or "God, I trust you," even when I wasn't quite sure if I really did. That was the start of the ever-growing relationship that I have with God today. It doesn't take much to begin, but it does take truly living in faith, not just in coming to believe.

The most common pushback to belief in God that I hear is that there are so many people who claim belief in God behaving in ways that are not aligned with unconditional love. From my experience, there are two possibilities here. One possibility is that they aren't perfect, and I need to cut them a break because I, too, am imperfect, even if it isn't in quite the same way that they are.

The second possibility, and the more likely possibility when the departure from unconditional love runs to extremes, is that you have found someone who believes in God, but who is not truly living in faith, not truly turning their will and their life over to the care of God. These individuals include a much larger number of believers than you might imagine.

They believe with their head that God exists, but they aren't living in faith. They aren't turning the care of their heart and mind over to God. As a result, they are not only suffering inside, but they also are often trying to outwardly control situations and other people. They think they know best and tell others what to do rather than loving them.

I used to make the mistake of believing that God was the problem. I now recognize it as a simple human problem, and I choose not to let someone else's behavioral manifestation of lack of faith lead me away from a life filled with divine love. My hope is that if people like this have left a bad taste in your mouth, you are able to understand the issue from this new perspective, offer them a little grace, and give God another shot.

The journey to faith is always available. Peace of soul is always available. Letting go of the need to control is always available. But it takes faith, not just belief.

Lesson 9

God Can Make Lemonade Out of Anything

On Christmas day in 2020, I met a man named Kevin. Although I didn't know it that day, I had met my future husband. We didn't start dating right away, in part because I had a boyfriend named Seth. A little over a week after I met Kevin, I broke up with Seth, and Kevin and I started spending more time together. I didn't know what God's plan was, and I barely believed in God at the time, but I did know something different than I had ever experienced was happening between us.

On January 13th, Kevin left on a motorcycle trip with a group of his friends. They hauled their motorcycles via trailer from Minnesota to Scottsdale, Arizona, and then took off toward Mexico from there. Their final destination was Mazatlán, Mexico. Kevin and I FaceTimed almost every day of his men-only trip, laughing and praying together on the phone. Then I got a call midday on January 19th from Kevin.

He told me that he had totaled his motorcycle and was going back to Arizona. He had been in the parking lot of their resort, showing his friends the sport mode on his new-to-him 2018 Honda Goldwing. He meant to do some kind of burnout, but the gear caught, and instead of the burnout, the motorcycle shot full speed across the parking lot and into the wheel well of a Hummer. The motorcycle was totaled. The Hummer had to be towed away because the impact had caused the tie rod to break. Kevin was lucky that the Hummer was parked where it was because behind the Hummer was a cement wall. The impact would have been a lot different had he hit the wall. The accident likely would have sent him to the hospital or even killed him.

That day, the hand of God on the whole incident was clear. Kevin was barely injured, except for a scrape on his chin and losing a flip flop, and he was already talking about the bright side of the incident, namely, that we could get to know each other on an impromptu trip. He was going to fly back to Arizona and wait for the guys. He invited me to fly down and spend a few days with him and then join him on the drive back to Minnesota. That trip to Arizona and the drive back changed my relationship not only with Kevin, but also with God. I was new to sobriety at the time, and for me, our journey was simultaneously God-centered sobriety bootcamp and getting to know someone who would turn out to be my future husband. That was enough to prove that God can make lemonade out of lemons. Kevin would never have wished for the crash to happen, but the resulting trip changed both of our lives.

However, the story does not end there. Three years later, Kevin and his friends left for their annual motorcycle trip. They planned to head to Cabo this time, but after looking at the weather, they decided they would go back to Mazatlán. After a few beautiful days of riding through the Sierra Madre mountains, they arrived in Mazatlán and decided to clean up their bikes. As they were washing their bikes, Kevin's friend Dave realized that the rear brake line on his motorcycle was broken off. "I wish I had never even seen that," Dave said. He knew repairing or replacing it would be tough in Mazatlán and almost wished he had just continued on his way, blissfully unaware of the damage. It's spooky to realize you have been riding without rear brakes, as is the prospect of riding a thousand miles back to Arizona through the mountains of Mexico without them.

They decided to find a motorcycle shop to see if there was anything that a local mechanic could do. They went to the nearest shop, and the shop owner looked at them with wide eyes. The largest bikes they sold and serviced at that time in Mazatlán were 650cc motorcycles, far smaller than the 1800cc massive Honda Goldwing touring bike that Dave was riding. There was no chance that the parts they had would work on Dave's motorcycle. The shop owner told them that the closest place that serviced motorcycles of that size was in a nearby major city—however, it was a city known for its cartel presence.

Just as they were about to give up, one of the mechanics who had been chatting with Kevin's friend, Patrick, said he might have an idea. He told Patrick to follow him to the back of the shop. Patrick did so, and then returning to the front, he signaled to Kevin to follow him into the back of the shop. Kevin described how Patrick had a sparkle in his eye that he had not seen before in their eighteen years of friendship. Kevin followed Patrick to the back of the shop, and all Dave could hear in the front was laughter—joyful astonishment and laughter because the problem had been solved.

Kevin's totaled 2018 Honda Goldwing was sitting in the back room of the shop, covered in dust. It had been towed there after the accident in 2021. Kevin had been mailed an insurance check and had turned the title over to the insurance company. Evidently, the insurance company had figured the bike was worthless and had decided just to leave it in Mexico. No one had ever communicated any of this to the shop owner, and he had never figured out what to do with it, so it had just been sitting for three years. What's more, Dave was riding a 2018 Honda Goldwing. Although Kevin's totaled Goldwing was damaged and had been sitting for three years, the brake lines were in perfect condition. Dave got the brake lines and ended up trading his windshield for the windshield on Kevin's old motorcycle. Patrick upgraded his bike's luggage rack with a trade for the one on Kevin's old motorcycle. The shop charged them only $45 for all the labor. There was no charge for the parts since the bike was Kevin's to begin with.

I can always use a reminder that God exists and that God can use all things for good, and I love a good story where these truths are glaring and undeniable. God can always do for me what I can't do for myself. God is always working, and I never know what surprise God has waiting for me around the corner.

Lesson 10

Trust That the Message Is from God

In April of 2022, I went on my first ever spiritual retreat. I had signed up for the retreat on a whim and convinced Kevin, my then boyfriend and now husband, to sign up as well. This retreat has taken place on a regular basis for years. I had heard about it sometime in early 2021, but for some reason, on April 5, 2022, I signed Kevin and me up for this weekend retreat, knowing almost nothing about it. All I knew was that we would head for the retreat on Saturday morning and return on Monday.

On Thursday, April 7, 2022, Randi, a close friend of mine, overdosed and died. When I found out that Thursday night, the retreat was the last thing on my mind; and when I woke up on Friday morning, I was questioning whether I should still go. The retreat was to be cell phone free, so going would mean I would not be able to make or receive calls or respond to messages from Saturday morning to Monday evening. I was a mentor to several women in recovery who were also close friends with Randi. Would it be unsupportive of me to go? Would I be abandoning them if I left to go on the retreat? Like any person of faith, I prayed for guidance, and I felt strongly that God was telling me I still ought to go to the retreat. Kevin and I arrived on Saturday morning, and I quickly dove into the retreat. This was a retreat specifically for first timers at this retreat center. I have not been to many adult retreats, but what became clear to me is that adults attending spiritual retreats for the first time often have something that they are going through, whether it is a recent happening or a longstanding existential crisis. Although

Randi's death was perhaps one of the most recent happenings that anyone at the retreat was working through, I fit right in.

During the retreat, we were each assigned to a small group of approximately six or seven people. Although Julia was not in my group, she caught my attention throughout the weekend because of her level of despair. She didn't stop crying the first day. I was sure things would be better for her by Sunday, but nothing had changed. By Sunday evening, it was clear that something was very wrong. In one of the sessions, she finally shared that she was grieving for her husband, who had passed away about a year prior to the retreat. He had been diagnosed with cancer early in 2021, and within a few months, he was dead. It had been a year since he had passed, but her emotions were still extremely raw.

As we entered one of the Sunday late night activities, I happened to be lined up behind her as we walked along a path and then were seated in a prayer circle. As we sat and she continued to sniffle, something came over me, and I knew that God was calling me into prayer. I closed my eyes and silently began to pray. I wasn't so much praying for any particular outcome or relief from grief for her. I can't really explain what happened, but I just knew I was supposed to get quiet. I began praying. I am not the sort of person who usually visualizes anything while praying, but suddenly in my mind's eye, I saw the color blue, then a sort of green, and then a pickup truck. I was confused, but the images were clear. This was odd. Then another feeling or thought came over me—I was supposed to tell Julia. That's where my ego began to take over. How was I supposed to tell her? What was I supposed to say? It would be too awkward. I'd had one short conversation with her earlier in the weekend, but with that exception, I had not talked with her much at all.

I ignored the message. We left prayer time and headed back to the main room, where we had one last activity before bedtime. As everyone was leaving the main room at bedtime, the feeling that I needed to deliver the message about my visual experience to Julia became so strong that it almost felt like anxiety. I knew I had to tell her. I walked over to her, tapped her on the shoulder, and said, "Julia, do you have a minute?" She replied, "Sure."

I continued, "So, this is not something I really know anything about, and I am not really sure why, but I was praying before when we were in the prayer circle, kind of for you, you know, just because you have been crying all weekend." (I know, foot in mouth moment.) "And so, um, well, I think I am supposed to tell you 'blue truck.' " She stared at me with a look I perceived to be confusion. I continued, "Never mind, I am not really sure…" She interrupted my rambling, "No, wait, what kind of truck?" I said, "I don't know car brands all that well." Not thinking about the fact that I hadn't described my vision at all and instead had just blurted out, "blue truck." She clarified, "No, I mean like a large semi-truck, pickup truck, dump truck, tow truck?" I replied, "Oh, of course, yes, a blue pickup truck." For the first time in the conversation, she looked interested, "What color blue? Like a turquoise?" My face lit up, "Oh! I actually saw blue and then green and then the truck, so maybe that's what that was!"

Then she just looked at me, stunned, and started crying. I wasn't sure what to do, and she wasn't sure either. After what felt like forever, she looked up and said, "Just before my husband's diagnosis, he bought a turquoise blue pickup truck to fix up to go fishing with my son. Then he got sick, and it never happened. But…I think, I think God is trying to tell me that my husband is with Him and he's okay." I gave her a long hug, and we parted for bedtime.

The next morning at breakfast she came over to me. Something was different, and she wasn't crying. She went on to tell me that she'd had the best night's sleep of any she'd had in months, and she had finally taken off her wedding ring. The peace stayed with her the rest of the day until the retreat ended. She thanked me again before leaving, even though we both knew it was God, not me. Two months later, we returned to the site of the retreat for a reunion. She came over to me and told me that the message I had taken the time to listen to that night had changed the course of her grief, and that she hadn't put her wedding ring back on. She knew her husband was at peace, and so was she. She had been able to return to actually living life.

I tell this story today as a reminder to slow down. God works in mysterious ways that we can't imagine. It has been more than three years since I delivered that message, and God has worked in many amazing ways in my life, but I will never forget that day. It is a reminder that when I get out of the way, God uses me as a channel of His divine plan and works miracles I could never orchestrate on my own. I know the same is true for every human on this Earth. When we get quiet enough and truly believe that anything is possible, suddenly anything *is* possible.

Lesson 11

Stop Praying That the World Changes

As a little girl, I had a prayer journal. I found that journal a few years ago, and it had some very specific requests. For example, burglars had recently broken into the garage at my dad's house several times, and I had requested that God please stop the burglaries. I remember learning about famine and the starving children in other countries and praying to God to stop the kids from starving. Although I do not remember it because I was so young, it would not be a stretch to guess that I probably prayed that my parents wouldn't get divorced or would change their minds about the divorce.

Although my prayers may have taken many forms, what these prayers all have in common is that they are requests to God to please stop "bad" things from happening. On the surface, these seem like reasonable requests, but are they? And what do they reveal about my faith? When I prayed those prayers, I was a child, so I will give myself a break in that regard, but is asking God to stop "bad" things from happening a reasonable request as an adult? I'll start by saying that if it is part of your prayers, this essay is not a pitch for you to stop, but instead the story of my waking up to the truth—for me—about prayers like these.

Like many misguided spiritual endeavors of my past, I have come to understand that the futility of prayers like these is that they are selfish. At face value, this may not seem to be the case, but a deeper dive begins to reveal that they are. I wanted the garage to stop being broken into because it made me scared. It also upset my dad and stepmom when it happened. Why do I care about that? Because when they are upset, I am not sure how to act, and I am uncomfortable. Interesting, that also appears to be about me.

But what about the children starving in Africa? Shouldn't I pray for them? I am not saying don't, but it is worth questioning my own motives. Is it because it makes me sad and uncomfortable that other kids are suffering or because I believe that it is inherently bad if they are suffering? What about my parents' divorce? It might be simpler to see how this one is selfish; I was mad that they were not together. It made me upset. It inconvenienced me. Other kids at school thought it was weird, and I had to deal with the consequences of that.

Me. Me. Me.

In each case, I placed myself at the center of the universe and decided that the universe was unfolding incorrectly, and so it needed to be changed. I decided that this or that must be "bad" because I was uncomfortable or someone else was uncomfortable, which ultimately made me uncomfortable.

Prayer, as I use it now, is never a request to stop "bad" things from happening. I do not pray selfish prayers. I pray to see things differently. I pray to see things as God sees them. I ask for direction or action if I am to take it. But I never pray to God so as to suggest that His plan is unfolding incorrectly.

So, instead of selfish prayers in hopes that the universe unfolds differently, my prayers to see the world differently help me to accept life on life's terms. My prayers stop me from making the misguided judgment that anything going on outside of me is inherently bad. When I decide that something is inherently bad, I am showing God that

I do not have faith in His power to use everything for good, and that I believe my feelings are more important than the unfolding of reality for the collective.

Before I had a relationship with God, things were bad when I decided they were bad. Today, I know better. I am responsible for not engaging in wrongdoing myself and for asking God to keep me from wrongdoing and the near occasion of wrongdoing, something I cannot do on my own. But I was not placed on this Earth to judge other people or situations as wrong. I was put here to ask God to help me do right, to follow His will for my life, to trust His plan, and to love others, no matter their actions.

When my prayers are focused on this, I do not sit around wallowing at what is going on in the world. I have faith that I won't ever be able to understand the vastness of God's plan, and that my job is to love people the best I can as that plan unfolds. After all, it's called the mystery of faith for a reason, and some of the greatest acts of love and of faith have come at the most difficult times. When I can remember life is not about me and not meant for me to understand, life goes a lot more smoothly.

PART II

Spiritual Diagnostics

Lesson 12

The Truth about Admitting Powerlessness

I used to struggle with admitting I was powerless. I couldn't understand why admitting powerlessness is the first step of so many addiction recovery programs. (I hope I don't lose those of you who are not in recovery, because the concept involved extends far beyond recovery from addictions, something that will become clear by the end of this essay.) Specifically, I couldn't understand why admitting powerlessness over alcohol was necessary for me to be able to stop drinking.

How does that make sense?

I felt as though I was being asked to admit that I was powerless over an inanimate object. I would sit there thinking, I am literally not powerless. I can smash it. I can burn it. I can pour it down the sink. I can throw it away. How could I be powerless over a bottle of alcohol? I had gone days without drinking before.

Didn't that prove I wasn't powerless? Never mind that I always used to start again.

Nevertheless, I conceded powerlessness, but not with any clear understanding of why. It was a good place to start. I was admitting that I didn't have the answers anymore. I could stop drinking, but I couldn't keep myself from starting again no matter how much I tried. I could see it in my other obsessions as well. I knew that no matter what I did, my eating disorder always seemed to somehow return. Sure, I guess that was powerlessness. I used to have some pretty intense OCD as a child that involved flicking light switches, and although that was mostly gone, it occasionally returned in short bouts as well. But why did I have to admit I was powerless over peanut butter, vodka, or light switches in order to recover? That was the part that made no sense.

As it turns out, I just had an elementary, perhaps even misguided, understanding of powerlessness. Today, I know that I am actually at my best, experiencing life to the fullest, when I admit that I am powerless over everything. This is one of the major paradoxes of life as I know it. The more I believe that I can and should control anything, the worse it goes and the more painful it feels in the long run. Ironically, the peak of this climb up the mountain of control was my rock bottom. Admitting powerlessness was an act of surrender as well as the first erosion of the mountain of control that was my suffering. Suffering comes from trying to control things that are not meant to be in my control.

So, I am powerless over alcohol and drugs. It turns out I am also powerless over my eating disorder. I am powerless over my OCD. I am powerless over anxiety. I am powerless over depression. I am powerless over dishonesty. I am powerless over pride. I am powerless over vanity and materialism. I am powerless over seeking approval from others, especially men. I am powerless over endless comparisons to others. I am powerless over financial insecurity. I am powerless over anger. I am powerless over fear. I am powerless over seeking validation on social media. The list could go on.

You know who isn't powerless over those things? God. You know why I now rarely struggle with most of the things on that list? Surprise! It is my relationship with a living God. Spoiler, God lives in you, too, whether you acknowledge it or not. And thus, the real story of recovery and of the mystery of faith begins to unfold. *It is only by turning to God and humbly admitting that I am powerless and need God's help that I get to experience lasting change.* When I tried to change any of those things with my human power, they sometimes changed, but only for a little while.

All you have to do is put someone trying to change their behavior using self-will under a little stress and their true colors are quickly revealed. They are powerless. Moreover, when you find someone who is stuck in self-willed behavior change, they aren't fun to be around. They are full of pride and believe that they are superior for doing what they are doing. They expect you do just grit your teeth and change, just the way they did. They generally won't hold your hand and help you succeed. When you find someone who has admitted they were powerless and turned their will over to God, they are helpful and humble. They want you to succeed.

They want to show you their path.

The beautiful thing that I have come to understand is that when I am willing to admit that I am powerless, I am ready to turn that area of my life—that behavior change—over to God. That's how things actually change in my life permanently and for the better, by an act of surrender and humility, not control and power. When I tried to stop drinking using my own will, I usually found myself full of anxiety and with an ever-worsening eating disorder. Clinicians like to refer to my predicament as cross-addiction, which it is. But what is cross-addiction? Cross-addiction is a phenomenon where when a person overcomes one addiction, they fall into another. Cross-addiction is the result of someone using self-will instead of surrender to change their behavior. Instead of "God, I surrender, show me the next step," it's "God, I got this, I already know the next step." These paths lead to very different long-term outcomes physically, psychologically, emotionally, and spiritually.

I sit here as someone with a PhD in psychology whose expertise is in behavior change, and I am telling you that my experience is that lasting behavior change in my life and in the lives of others I have witnessed—lasting behavior change that turns into an effortless part of someone's life—has only ever come by surrender to a Higher Power, whom I call God. So, I no longer struggle to admit that I am indeed powerless over everything, and I hope someday you realize you are, too.

Lesson 13

The Opposite of Addiction Is Not Connection

There is a now infamous Technology, Education, Design talk (TED talk) called, "Everything You Think You Know about Addiction is Wrong." In it, Johann Hari challenges the idea that addiction is tied to chemical hooks which ultimately alter an addict's neurochemical balance, leading to addiction to the chemical. He cites a plethora of evidence that makes a lot of sense. For example, 20 percent of troops during the Vietnam War were using heroin, leading to concern that large numbers of troops would return home as addicts. However, 95 percent of the troops who came home stopped using it. Relatedly, I used to believe that I had a physical allergy to alcohol rather than a spiritual malady. That fell apart when I realized that ripe bananas, brioche bread, and yogurt all contain alcohol. Yet, there was no addiction or allergic reaction to these foods. If you want more on why addiction is not really just about chemical hooks, google his TED talk. I am on board. Addiction is not just chemical hooks and brain chemistry.

Next, Hari goes on to propose that addiction is really about an addict's environment and surroundings, and famously, that the opposite of addiction is connection. His proposition is based on the "Rat Park Experiment." Here is how it goes. If you put a rat alone in a cage and give it water or a drug cocktail, the rat not only chooses the drug cocktail but drinks it until it overdoses and dies. If you instead put rats in a "rat park," a large cage with food, toys, and other rats to play and mate with, the rats mostly just choose water, and none of them use the drug cocktail to excess. He concludes that the opposite of addiction is connection, that addicts just need different surroundings, a purpose in life, closer friends, better toys, maybe a loving partner, you name it. He ends by saying that he now sits on addicts' couches and makes sure they know that he loves them whether they are using or not.

Here is what Hari missed. Rats don't have a conscience the way humans do. Rats aren't suffering from past wounds or future anxieties. They aren't struggling with a recent break-up or fearfully standing on the side of the road because their car just broke down. They aren't grieving a loss from years ago. They aren't jealous of their successful sister. They aren't angry about betrayal. They aren't afraid that their partner will leave them. They don't wish they were as skinny as their best friend. They aren't suffering from anxiety about whether Sally Rat likes them. Rats don't feel alone in a crowded room because they are "too in their head." If there is a playground, they play.

As an addict, I have had the experience of being in a proverbial "rat park" with people around me showing me love in any number of ways, and still not feeling "a part of." Using solves it. I have been caught in grief. Using solves it. I have been unable to let go of the shame of past mistakes. Using solves it. I have had the experience of hating and obsessing about my body. Using solves it. I have had the feeling of not being able to let go of blame and unforgiveness. Using solves it. I have had fear about the future. Using solves it. As a result of the state of my internal world, there was a 100 percent chance that Lisa of the past would use to excess no matter how supportive the "rat park" of loved ones connected to me at the time.

In the words of mindfulness teacher Jon Kabat-Zinn, "Wherever you go, there you are." And as long as I was there with an unexamined conscience, I was there with a deep-seated notion of separation, regardless of the "rat park" or loving human connections around me.

The opposite of addiction, as I have experienced it, is not connection. My addiction was never solved by someone sitting on my couch and telling me that they love me regardless of whether I choose to use or not. In real life, people actually do this a lot more than Hari seems to realize; and although it feels good in the short term, and sometimes tears of relief are even shed, I have yet to see it produce lasting change.

That is because the opposite of addiction is not connection with others, it is internal peace, peace of soul. It's an inside job. It is available to me alone in a cell or in the presence of other humans, and it isn't about others loving me more or in the right way. Feeling better because I get more love from others or get love the way I want it is attachment, not freedom. Peace of soul rests on whether I am willing to do the internal work, not whether you can show me love in the right way, and that is actually the gift of it. It's all up to me.

As I sit here writing this, I can tell you that for me, the solution to addiction was not to change the conditions of my life, make new friends, move to a new city, get closer connections, or be with my loved ones, in other words, to find my "rat park." That is because my problem wasn't lack of connection, my problem was that, unbeknownst to those around me, I was so uncomfortable in my skin, so full of confusion floating around in my unexamined conscience, that I couldn't even experience the love sitting right in front of me.

Therefore, the solution for me was to do the work to examine my conscience and find all the pain in there, ranging from resentment and fear to jealousy and judgment, and to blaming others for the present pain of past wounds. Freedom from all this relieved the uncomfortable feelings of despair, anxiety, worry, shame, remorse, and regret, to name a few, feelings that I not only used to suffer from but that also inevitably led to the need to use (alcohol, drugs, food, men, etc.). In the wake of this work, I found peace of soul, the true opposite of addiction and the condition in which using doesn't cross my mind nor show up in my dreams.

Although I barely believed in the power of prayer at the start of doing this work, I ended up needing a whole lot of it to examine my conscience, let go of my pain, and experience true peace of soul. Only you know if you need it, too. In short, freedom from addiction didn't result from connection or changing any of the other conditions of my life, it came about from allowing change to the condition of my soul, so that I can live at peace, free from addiction, regardless of the conditions of my life. Hari is welcome on my couch any time, but my recovery doesn't depend on it, and that's actually a blessing.

Lesson 14

Another Day of Sobriety Is the Wrong Goal

I was once listening to a recovery speaker who was able to put words to something that I have understood for a long time but had not articulated in quite this way. In short, he said that sobriety should not be the goal of recovery.

At face value, this seems like an odd statement. I thought I was in recovery to get sober. I thought sobriety would start to solve the problems piling up in my life. For those who were just drinking a little too much, but not compulsively or "alcoholically," it seems that sobriety is a worthwhile goal. Some of these people may even call themselves alcoholics or have gone to treatment. But here's the acid test: When these people stop drinking, their life gets better. Their mood improves. They sleep better. They save money. This essay isn't for them. This essay is for people like me. And when I stopped drinking, my life did not effortlessly get better.

For the record, I have no problem with the segment of the sober community that fits the above description, but it can be confusing for someone like me, who drank compulsively and had a very different experience of not drinking. When I stopped drinking, other people suffered less because I stopped causing them anxiety; but I lost my number one way of coping with life, namely drinking, and my life did not get better at that point.

I felt the emotions I had been avoiding for years. I felt anxious; I felt angry; I felt miserable; I felt pain that I couldn't describe. I would fall into despair, often diagnosed as clinical depression, but it was really just the opposite end of the restlessness and irritability I was experiencing that was sapping my whole body of energy. I said I was doing okay with sobriety, that things were getting better, but inside, things were feeling more confusing than ever.

For people like me, sobriety can become a dangerous goal because it gets so many people off track. If I stop drinking and I am still anxious, still depressed, and still can't handle life on life's terms, and sobriety is my only goal, I may try to achieve that goal in any number of ways that do not address the root problem. One direction might be prescription medications like Inderal, Xanax, Lexapro, or Zoloft, or perhaps relegating myself to being California sober, that is, using cannabis only. Another avenue might be endless consumption of energy drinks. Maybe I choose methadone or suboxone. Maybe I try to fill my time and social life with sober bowling leagues or more sober social events. Maybe I start reading more or watching more Netflix. Maybe I pick up new hobbies to stay busy or put in more hours at work. Maybe I just attend recovery meeting after recovery meeting.

All those avenues, some fun and healthy, some not so fun or healthy, were ways I tried or thought about trying in order to try to pass time so that I didn't drink for another day. None of these ever produced anything except one more day to add to a sobriety day count. What was I hoping I would gain by making it through another day? Perhaps that a magic number of sober days would take away the pain I was experiencing.

The magic number of days never came, and I did not think it was ever going to come. That is the problem with sobriety time as a goal. It is a bit like an employer who is frustrated by lack of productivity, so he says that all employees must be in the office forty hours a week. What he can be sure of is that people will be in the office forty hours per week. Will this increase productivity? Most likely not, because the goal has nothing to do with the real problem. The real problem is productivity.

For people like me, the real problem isn't that I needed more sober days, it's that I did not know how to live in peace with others and enjoy the big and small moments in life. I did not know how to cope with life on life's terms. So, when my main goal was to stay sober another day, I could use any means to do that, but most means of doing that do not address the root spiritual problem.

Lack of sobriety was never the problem; the problem was lack of spiritual awakening—living asleep was the problem. Therefore, sobriety should not be the goal. When sobriety is the goal, anything can be the means. When a spiritual awakening that puts me in a position of neutrality around alcohol and drugs is the goal, the way is narrow, but the fruits are the fruits of the spirit, not another day of avoiding my emotions that happens to count toward my sober day count. When the goal is spiritual awakening, the means has to be seeking God, and when my goal became seeking God instead of staying sober, my whole life changed.

Lesson 15

Self-Control Won't Keep Me Sober

My eyes opened. It was April 22, 2020, at 6:30 a.m. Although it was still dark outside, I had left the light on in my apartment, stinging my eyes as they opened. I suddenly realized I could feel the sticky wet sheets beneath me. "Not again," I thought. I had gotten white sheets for this apartment, determined that my drinking would be over this time, with the pristine white signifying the purity of this new phase of life. The white was now stained not only with urine and sweat, but also with blood from my favorite monthly visitor. I sat up and realized one of the plastic risers had slipped out from under my bed frame, leaving the bed at a tilt.

Good morning to me, my blood- and urine-stained sheets, and my crooked bed. At least it made it easier to roll out and onto my feet. *I could barely stand the smell of myself.* Without even thinking, I walked over to the fridge, and to my dismay, found my only alcoholic drink option to be a box of red wine. "Whatever, this will do." I squirted myself a glass from the tiny valve. I choked as I took the first few sips, and then added a splash of kombucha to soften the harsh flavor and to make it more of a breakfast drink as well as make myself believe my situation wasn't so dire. I quickly chugged down the now slightly fizzy cocktail and collapsed onto the couch. At least I can't hear my heartbeat in my head anymore, I thought as I laid there.

I thought I just needed more self-control. Why couldn't I just stop? Why couldn't I just change my behavior? I use this example only because of the extremity of the self-control issue I faced. No matter how much

I tried, how many reasons I had, how many rules and boundaries I set, I couldn't stop drinking. Moreover, I couldn't understand why I had no self-control. At the time the story I just told took place, I was a postdoctoral fellow in the Department of Preventive Medicine at Northwestern University School of Medicine. I had a PhD in psychology, and the focus of my studies had been behavior change. I knew it all—all the theories and all the tricks—and yet I couldn't change my own behavior. I just couldn't muster the self-control I needed for this one.

As it turns out, that is because self-control wasn't the solution. That was my biggest mistake. Sitting here writing this, I haven't had a drink in more than three years, and I don't struggle to avoid it. Self-control is not part of the equation, nor is any behavior change theory. Instead, my ability to experience this radical change in behavior was contingent on my capacity to drop my pride enough to believe that there might be another way, free of plans and resolutions.

This new way required following those who had gone before me into the Great Unknown, because it turns out the key to behavior change is thorough introspection—truly deep and thorough introspection.

Those who had gone before me showed me that truly thorough introspection, deep soul-searching if you will, requires God's assistance, and it took some time for me to come to believe it and experience it. However, to this day, I can't access my conscience at the depth that I need to without God's assistance. This is because thorough introspection not only requires that I find the parts of myself I would rather not seek out, or perhaps barely have awareness of, but also that I fully understand and admit that I am the sole cause of these parts. No one else is to blame. What kinds of parts? Resentment, jealousy, judgment, financial insecurity, body image obsession, and self-pity, to name a few.

Why would I do this? Because when I have nothing in my conscience left to avoid, I have no reason to engage in any escapism, and as it turns out, I don't think about drinking. It literally doesn't cross my mind.

Easier said than done? For sure. It requires looking at myself in ways that are painful and confusing as I unearth these parts. I used to have too much pride to even begin the process, let alone admit that the path requires God's assistance. But my experience has been that the reward for engaging in thorough introspection is the absence of the need for self-control.

This applies not only to my use of alcohol and drugs, but also to how how I eat, how I move, what I buy, how I treat others, my anxiety, and my anger. In short, it applies to how I show up in my life. Formerly baffling and seemingly uncontrollable cycles I used to be stuck in are now in control, without an ounce of self-control.

Lesson 16

How to Avoid Consenting to Cravings

I was walking on the treadmill when I suddenly felt discomfort. It wasn't related to walking; it was as though a general anxiety was creeping over me. Then the thoughts came. "Maybe just stop. Ten minutes is good for today. Maybe go home and jump on the trampoline for ten minutes if twenty minutes is your goal." As that thought crossed my mind, an image of the kitchen flashed through my mind. Then, my mind started racing, scanning for possible snacks. I had eaten lunch. It was not yet dinner time. Nutritionally, I did not need a snack, but that didn't stop my mind from trying to convince me that I did—that I should just go home. I knew that if I went home at that moment, it would only make me annoyed at myself, for behaving like a quitter. "Maybe I can stay on the treadmill and meditate for ten minutes." I pushed all the thoughts away, barely acknowledging the sense of craving at hand, but I couldn't seem to meditate.

After twenty minutes of walking, I left and went to my car. Immediately, my brain thought, "Maybe have a pack of Mentos mints when you get home. What is the plan for dinner? Maybe a snack now, and then just have less at dinner." Other ideas started racing through. "Maybe just a spoonful of probiotic yogurt. Maybe a spinach wrap. Maybe something small." Suddenly my mind was full of thoughts, and my body was full of an uncomfortable anxious feeling. My mind was racing so fast that I could barely keep up with it.

I know that if my mind starts racing too fast, somehow my body will make it to the kitchen and begin snacking. It won't be a reasonable snack, though; it will snowball into something else completely, more than likely to the tune of at least a few thousand calories—a binge. Then I will feel full and gassy and consider purging. I may even start obsessing about the gym—whether I should have gone—as I relapse into the belief that the gym is a place to burn calories rather than a place to get healthier. I might even fear that all the carbs I just ate will bloat my muscles and make it worse. I'll consider laxatives or an overdose of magnesium. I will consider how uncomfortable it will be to try to show up for any social plans I have for the night.

If I start the binge, I won't be able to stop. I will ruin dinner with my husband, and I will have to tell him what happened, or else be too embarrassed to tell him and instead just stuff dinner on top, become even more uncomfortably full, and then tell him I am super tired and go to bed right away when we get home—while hoping I am not too gassy overnight. I might even somehow try to sneak away from him to purge, but the length of the drawn-out binge will make it almost impossible to actually purge anything, and then I'll just be uncomfortably full and have indigestion.

If you have never had an experience like this with food, alcohol, drugs, shopping, or anything else, consider that a gift. You might ask, all that starts with a single uncomfortable feeling? Yes, that's a craving. That's not the craving of an everyday overeater or a casual drinker, that is the craving of someone with a compulsion. As a society, we sometimes understand such compulsions better when the drug of choice is alcohol or pills rather than food, but still not always. And equally important, some people find it all the more baffling when it's food, a substance that so many people can handle responsibly without any need for a spiritual program or awakening. If you're like me, I couldn't do it alone. I could hear the food calling to me, and renouncing it only made it louder. The same was true for alcohol. I am the type of person for whom normal psychological treatment programs, cognitive behavioral tools, or challenges like sober October just don't work. I needed something deeper.

Today, I have tools, the first of which I am going to make use of right now, because believe it or not, I wrote this essay in real time. My mind was racing, and I thought to myself, capture it. This may be the writer's version of the crying videos that influencers post on social media. In fact, I feel as though I might better understand the pause that they take to turn on the camera when they are having a meltdown, because something told me to take this pause and just write it out. I will be back after a short self-examination.

Welcome back. About twenty minutes before the craving began, my husband called to update me on some aspects related to his child custody case. He has a nine-year-old son whom I have never met due to a very messy divorce. I got confused near the end of the conversation with my husband and believed he might have been misinterpreting something. But, more than that, I didn't pray when the phone call ended. I just moved to the next thing. And when a person stays confused, they end up angry. Think about the last time you couldn't find something you were looking for, maybe a document, an invitation, or even your glasses or keys. At first, you were just confused, but if you remain confused for a few minutes, in a short time, you usually end up angry.

Anyway, I let my confusion fester. I was angry and fearful, because, of course, we are never so fearful as when we are angry. The biggest fear I could identify was that Kevin could be disappointed by the outcome of the next stage of the case. Some people would call that loving, but

I know better. It is attachment, not love, because I am making my emotions dependent on his. So, I prayed, "God, please forgive me for any judgment I had of Kevin's ability to understand the case and any fear I have about the case, my expectations, and Kevin's expectations. I know it is all in your hands and not for me to worry about or try to control."

As I finished praying and writing out the prayer, I can report that the craving has passed. Sometimes it takes longer. Sometimes it takes more prayers. Sometimes today's problems are just the visible problems and what I really need to get to are the root problems that require deeper examination. But, for today, I am thankful for God, for the peace I am now experiencing, and for God's nudge to write this all down in real time. Shallow recovery might tell you otherwise, but those of us who have had to go deep know that a craving is always caused by a separation from God, and the solution is always union with God through self-examination. It's deep. It's simple, yet not easy. It's spiritual. And if you're facing any addiction, it's also probably exactly what you need to hear.

Lesson 17

The Reality of Cross-Addiction

Although I don't remember how it all began, by the summer after my freshman year of high school, I was immersed in controlling food, exercise, and my body. I know some people have a particular moment when their eating disorder started. Maybe they binged after some type of stressful incident and felt relief or got approval for being thin or losing weight and felt belonging for the first time in their life. I don't remember any particular moment, but I do remember slowly sliding deeper and deeper into obsession throughout that summer.

By the fall of my sophomore year in high school, I had developed a full-blown eating disorder. Instead of me controlling my body, the eating disorder obsession now controlled me. I remember asking to use the restrooms during class and walking the halls of my school counting my steps. I stopped buying snacks and started repeating the phrase, "I am not really hungry," more than I ever had in my life. I started lying about food and manipulating meals to eat as little as possible while appearing normal. I would buy a turkey and cheese sandwich for lunch, but then I would walk down the hallway and throw away everything but a single slice of turkey. I would fill my bowl of Kashi Go Lean cereal with water, then add a splash of milk to make it appear white so people wouldn't question me. I took up running and called it a hobby. My brain was constantly calculating calories in and calories out.

Five months into my eating disorder, I was caught. I was 5'3" and weighed less than ninety pounds. I was sent to a dietician and a therapist. I was fifteen years old. The only time I ate normal food was when I was drunk, which was not a sustainable solution, especially since I blacked out almost every time that I drank, budding alcoholic that I was. By senior year of high school, I had restored my body to a normal weight. But nothing inside had been restored despite constant therapy.

For the next fifteen years, I shifted from eating disorder to eating disorder until I had been diagnosed with every eating disorder in the book. I went through phases of anorexia, marked by classic calorie restriction; phases of binge eating disorder marked by huge binges of thousands of calories without any particular purge, which not surprisingly led to very speedy weight gain; phases of exercise bulimia during which I made up for the calories I consumed through excessive and obsessive exercising; and phases of classic bulimia during which I purged through vomiting and laxative abuse. I always had a new pill, a new food that was off limits, a new diet I was secretly trying, or a new fast I was secretly going on. In the early 2000s, I was deeply enmeshed in the pages of eating disorder Tumblr blogs of the time. I was constantly lying about what and when I had eaten as well as hiding and even stealing food. If you asked me about what was on my plate, I would have a complete meltdown because I feared being seen and being caught.

The only commonality between all phases of the eating disorder was this: my brain was absolutely consumed by thinking about food, exercise, or body image related content. Period. The calculator was constantly running. I was obsessed. Sometimes I was fooling myself into thinking it was a hobby, sometimes I was in mild pain or anxiety about it, sometimes I was in deep despair, and sometimes I was relieved after weight loss or a purge. But almost always, my mind was consumed by eating-disorder-related thoughts. Sometimes my mind was fully consumed, sometimes it was more of a background noise, but it was almost always there—for fifteen years.

That is the key to what an eating disorder is. It is addiction—just like alcohol, like drugs, like codependency. As an alcoholic, I can tell you that thinking about and planning when to drink was just like an eating disorder. As an addict, I can tell you the same is true of drugs. As someone who used to be codependently obsessed with male approval, it's also the same. The beauty of it all? It meant that the resolution to my eating disorder was the same as for my alcoholism, drug addiction, and codependency. In the end, an eating disorder is just an obsession of the mind, same as any other addiction. There is nothing genetically wrong with me. There was never anything organically wrong with me. I just couldn't face the reality of my life, and so the obsession of the mind took over, in its many manifestations—cross-addictions galore.

There were cross-addictions galore in my life that all required but one single solution. Relief from the obsession of any addiction doesn't come from avoiding the thing in question nor from abstinence, relief comes from conscious contact with God. The path to that contact is to clear away what is blocking me from God—which takes a level of honesty that is quite difficult for most people, especially those currently caught in an obsession of the mind. If I don't have conscious contact with God, I'll end up with a cross-addiction. If I do, I won't.

When I can be rigorously honest with myself about the resentments and confusion I carry about my past and the anxiety I hold about my future, and truly turn those over to God, the addictions fall away. If I can't be honest with myself and with God about those things, the addictions remain because the obsession bubbles up as a means to avoid the simmering pain inside of me. It's a tough pill to swallow (pun intended), but it is the truth that has unfolded in my life. And just to be clear, the compulsive behavior simply follows the obsession of the mind. Drinking, drug use, eating, starvation, another relationship—they are all but symptoms of the obsession.

I never thought that I would be able to say that I understand my eating disorders, how I used to drink, the way I used drugs, or my compulsive dating life, but my experience has revealed to me that they are just a few manifestations of the same internal battle. When I honestly admit to the battles inside of me and turn them over to God, I have no use for an obsession.

Rigorous honesty with self and God is simple, but it is not easy. But, to start, as I sit here today in summer of 2024, I can tell you that for today, my calculator is off because of my connection with God. I am in a position of neutrality around food, exercise, and my body. I don't obsess about what or when I eat. The same goes for exercise. I don't obsess about how my clothes fit. I don't obsess about other people's weight. I don't try new diets. I don't have foods that are off limits. Resolving stress either by not eating, binge eating, or purging does not even come to mind anymore. I also don't think about drinking or using drugs. I don't obsess about men that I meet. I no longer engage in flirting. I don't imagine my life with other partners. I don't have to battle those thoughts. The battle is over. The battle isn't over because I tried to change those behaviors. The battle is over because I admitted I was wrong over and over again to God, to myself, and to another human being. So, for today, my spirit is free, and as such, I am free from obsessions.

Lesson 18

I Can't Change My Own Patterns

One of the hardest truths to swallow in my whole spiritual journey has been the truth that I cannot change myself. That may sound odd coming from someone whose life looks vastly different than it did a few years ago. I used to drink, and now I don't. The same is true for my use of street drugs, psychiatric prescription drugs, starving, binging, and most recently, consuming caffeine. In psychology, they might call these cross-addictions.

What's more fascinating is there are other aspects of my life that have dramatically changed. I used to spend hours shopping, both online and in person. I still shop, but the compulsion is not the same. I used to spend a lot of mental energy making sure everyone liked me; that too is less. I used to be crippled by financial fears and concerns, and I have somehow begun to let go of those. I used to think I couldn't eat a variety of foods, such as gluten and dairy. Now I eat all food groups. I used to wait to do everything until the last minute, while now I get most things done long before deadlines. I used to dress to attract men—or at the very least make sure my body was strategically seen. Yes, of course, I would tell you that it was for me and not for them, but deep down, I always knew I was lying to myself. How could I be getting dressed for myself when I was that absorbed in other people's opinions of me? The list goes on.

What is interesting about each of these changes is that I can't take any credit for them. Some of them I didn't even realize I was trying to change. Others I had been trying to change for years on my own yet had gotten nowhere. I had moments, even some long moments, of what I thought was relief, but always returned to the same behavioral prison.

By the time I had finished my PhD in psychology in 2019, while still drinking almost daily and still completely enmeshed in my eating disorder, I knew that behavior change theory offered little in the way of solutions to permanently change these behaviors. The focus of my PhD had been behavior change, and yet, there I was. It's not that behavior change theory has nothing to offer, but it has nothing to offer when the root of the problem is spiritual—as it was for me. Only you know whether this is the root of the problem for your behavior. The best way to find out is to try to change it yourself. If you consistently fail, the problem isn't the theory, the problem is that the difficulty at issue isn't behavioral. The symptom is behavioral, but the problem is spiritual. For the record, almost every problem behavior in my life was indeed spiritual in nature.

One of the key barriers I experienced in changing these behaviors is the influx of psychology into spirituality today, especially in recovery programs. People claim to be spiritual mentors, but they are teaching psychological principles to renounce behavior, an approach which only increased my spiritual tie to the problem behaviors. In spirituality, when I renounce, I give the problem power.

So, how did all these changes happen?

I let go. I surrendered. I asked God to do it. If you have tried this, you are probably relieved to see these words.

If you have not, you were probably looking for some fancy solution or actionable insight. This is because many of us have been so programmed to believe that we needed to try harder and do more, when all we needed to do was surrender.

What did surrender look like? First, I had to clear my conscience. This step assumes that I have done my best to remove the blocks between myself and God. The largest of these blocks are usually resentment and fear. Then, here is the actionable behavior. God doesn't decide what behaviors I am willing to see as problem behaviors—I must do that part. I had to see that I couldn't stop drinking, that I was consumed by people-pleasing, that I shopped all the time, that I was seeking approval from men, that I was jealous I did not have the financial freedom others had, and that I procrastinated. I had to not only see the pattern but also admit to God that I needed His help.

This is where the miracles happen. I have watched so many of my problematic habits fall away by this process, not always overnight, but some seemingly overnight. The hardest part of the process is truly letting go and trusting God. If I am still asking myself who I will be if I can't shop, people please, dress the way I did, or let go of control over my eating, the behavior won't go away because I am not ready to surrender. But, when I say, okay God, I am ready, it is just wild to watch how the behavior begins to fall away.

Lesson 19

Some People Don't Have to Go as Deep

I recently sat down with someone I am mentoring in sobriety and asked her how she was doing. She said she was good, but she looked like she would have crawled out of her skin if that had been a biological possibility. She is not brand-new. She is in what some refer to as the maintenance part of recovery, but it was clear that her spirituality was not being well-maintained. I answered her "Good," with, "I don't think you're actually good." She melted, metaphorically. She was not good. She couldn't pinpoint what was wrong, but I could—because I had been right where she was.

She agreed that restless, irritable, and discontent summed it up well. A short conversation revealed that she had done little to no self-examination nor prayer in weeks. I said, "Well, it would be surprising if you didn't feel irritable without prayer for this long. In fact, if you could just not do spiritual work for weeks and not suffer at all, you probably wouldn't have used alcohol to the extremes that you did, and you wouldn't need a sobriety mentor." We both laughed.

Walking away from the conversation, I reflected on various aspects of recovery that can make it extremely difficult, and one stood out to me. Namely, there are a lot of people who end up in recovery for any number of reasons and are able to go about their lives with little to no spiritual work and not relapse. Unfortunately, this can make it difficult for others who, like me and my mentee, suffer in the absence of daily self-examination and prayer.

This is not to suggest that those who do not engage in daily self-examination and prayer and manage to stay sober should leave the rooms of recovery. If that is you, I am happy you are sober if you are happy. I am happy to have you at recovery barbecues and get-togethers, planning trips and retreats, and in recovery meetings. Anyone with a desire to stop drinking or using is welcome in any recovery room.

My point is that what I see over and over again is that these individuals can be a poor model for those who, like me, are in need of a spiritual awakening to be sober, happy, joyous, and free. This is because it gives people like me the idea that conscious contact with God is not necessary for me to recover because this or that other person didn't need it. Perhaps more importantly, when these individuals try to mentor people like me, those who do need to surrender everything to God on a continual basis to stop suffering, one of two things happens: 1) the mentee never does deep spiritual work and continues to suffer for years while remaining abstinent from drugs and alcohol, or 2) the mentee finally suffers enough that they throw in the towel completely, believing that nothing will ever work.

In fact, in my heart of hearts, I know that wet houses, facilities where chronic alcoholics can be housed while they drink as much as they want, often to their grave, are full of people like me whose sole contact with recovery mentorship was someone who could not carry the depth of message they needed to recover. This is not because they did not want to carry a deeper message, but because they never needed that level of recovery themselves.

When I met my first recovery mentor, she had ten years of abstinence. She got sober at twenty-one after a DUI. At ten years of abstinence, she still had deep resentment against her mother, whom she had chosen not to forgive, and she told me that I could similarly hang onto resentment. When I wrote out my lifelong moral inventory, it read more as an inventory of my anger and other people's wrongs than a confession. I did not pray but once or twice during the whole process. My recovery mentor did not know any better. That is how she had done it. That's how her mentor had done it.

After six months of working with her and completion of a moral inventory without prayer, I started having daily anxiety attacks. Things were not better. I was still suffering. Luckily, I met someone who had done deeper spiritual work relating to recovery, not because he was better than anyone else, but because it was the only way he found sobriety and relief from suffering. He asked me how much prayer I had done. I told him little to none. He asked if I realized that my anger and unforgiveness toward others were wrongs that I had committed against my Creator. I said I had no idea.

He taught me to pray until I had forgiven everyone I had ever resented and to understand that I suffered from my own anger and unforgiveness, not from anyone else's behavior. He taught me how to go to God for help to understand the true nature of my behavior, and it became clear to me that I had created most of the suffering that I had endured through my own selfishness. He taught me how to examine myself whenever I am disturbed and turn what I find over to God.

Once I brought God into that lifelong moral inventory the way my new mentor had showed me, I experienced peace for the first time in my life. I also had the tools to repeat the process whenever a new disturbance arose. To this day, I have to repeat this process of self-examination and prayer every single day; otherwise, at best, I start to again become restless, irritable, and discontent, and at worst, the obsession with drink could begin to creep back in if I allowed myself to become increasingly disconnected from God.

Mentors who have had to go this deep themselves are the only ones who have the capacity to take others this deep. Mentors who can carry on with life without doing deep spiritual work are welcome in recovery. However, if you are being mentored by one of these well-meaning individuals and you are still suffering, please know that you are not alone and that there is help for you. In a few short months of working with a mentor who had truly given their life over to God and continued to do so on a daily basis, my life changed in ways that I never could have imagined. It just turns out I needed deeper work and could only be helped by a mentor who had done that level of work.

Lesson 20

I Was Addicted to Approval from Others

Letting go is not something that comes naturally to me. That may be why I spent so much time either tightly wound or blacked out. As a child, it was important to me to be right. As a young adult, it was important to me to be MVP in sports and get A's in school. In my twenties, it was important to me to appear intelligent to the other upper-middle class intellectuals with whom I spent time during the day and to appear attractive and successful to the wealthy, edgy, rebels with whom I spent time at night. I had unconsciously created several versions of myself that were carefully curated for whomever I was trying to impress at a given moment.

I often conducted my portrayal of these characters well enough to get quite a bit of approval from others. However, at times, the characters became unwound, especially late at night. More importantly, when alone, I felt uncomfortable and confused. I no longer had anyone to impress. I was lost. In the midst of it, if you had asked me whether I was playing a character, I would have either been overly nice to you to cover up the fact that I was offended or else I would have rolled my eyes and then complained about you to my friends to make sure that my ego could remain intact. My programming was strong enough that the journey away from a life of curation and calculation was not an easy one. The first step was to realize that I was living my life that way.

That only happened when I had finally had enough. I was exhausted. I had been playing games with eating and exercising for years in order to maintain a certain socially acceptable size. I carefully selected outfits for each of my characters, even when I appeared disheveled. I had earned a doctoral degree, the highest degree available. I had an important title at work. I meditated and subscribed to modern, new age, spiritual principles like manifesting abundance. I was dating wealthy entrepreneurs. I had curated my body, mind, spirit, and relationships. However, I was more confused and drinking more than ever. I did not know who I was or where I was going. Everything was externalized, subconsciously curated to impress others.

And luckily—yes, now I think it was lucky—I hit an emotional rock bottom. Over the three years since that rock bottom moment, I have realized that my most insidious problem and most longstanding addiction was to approval. I was constantly trying to do what everyone else wanted me to do. That's not people-pleasing. I am not a martyr. That is approval seeking. If you think you are a people-pleaser, I challenge you to examine yourself until you find out that pleasing others is actually seeking approval for yourself.

The greatest freedom I have found in the past three years is releasing and dropping the need for approval from others. That does not mean being a person who proclaims that they do not care what people think, it means actually being one. In fact, if you say aloud, "I don't give a s***" what other people think," I can almost guarantee that you care so much that you need to prove to others that you do not care by saying it aloud. To the contrary, I fully accepted that I was totally obsessed with trying to seek approval from others, and I began to ask God for help.

The result has been an incredible journey of seeing just how addicted I was to approval and finally watching it begin to fall away. This is not a decision from the mind that "I don't give a s***;" instead, I watched my thoughts, emotions, actions, and beliefs about life shift and change before my eyes. The deeper I leaned into seeking God's help, the more my former programming seemed to fall away. Time and time again, situations have come up in which I could feel that I was losing societal approval. Each and every time, I turned to God, and I was able to comfortably let the need for approval slip away. At first it was difficult, partially because it took praying to a God that I barely believed in. But over time, it has gotten easier and easier as I trust God more and more to guide me through each and every situation.

Today, I am somewhere between unemployed and starting a small business. Half the people I talk to about the business think I am joking, and yet I feel called to pursue it. I know it will be a success as long as I am not attached to what success means, because money or no money, I am going in the direction God appears to be pointing me. I won't be using my doctoral degree at all for the time being. I married a man without a college degree, a sober alcoholic who has been married twice before. I got a motorcycle license and I now ride motorcycles, despite fear of disapproval from my family and certain friends. I go into public all the time makeup free, a near impossibility a few years ago unless I was in a hungover, "I don't give a s***," kind of mood. I talk about God, not just the universe. I regularly tell stories about the darkest parts of my past to help others, and I readily tell people I am an alcoholic and an addict and that I have eating disorders.

Yet I am happier than ever, because except when God takes over and starts compelling me to write an essay like this, I don't even think about what my life looks like today. I just experience it. I feel called here or there, and I go, I do. I sign up for things. I experience things. I laugh with my friends. I eat. I listen to music. I just enjoy life. I do not try to manifest or pray for certain jobs, homes, friends, or outcomes, because when someone is truly happy, that literally does not even make sense. When I was stuck in craving approval as my source of happiness, however, it made all the sense in the world.

I do not ever really know what I am going to do or what's next, or what turns life might take, but I know that life is supposed to be this, not a game of seeking approval. This is letting go as I experience it today, and although I cannot tell you what's next, I can tell you that it will be just what it is supposed to be.

Lesson 21

I Thought I Was a People-Pleaser

I said, "I don't know what to say, I'm a people-pleaser," defending my behavior as I explained it to my therapist. She lovingly shook her head, as is her job, and said, "I understand that desire to be loved by others." She was helping me feel better, but she didn't understand the debilitating fear that was lurking underneath my people-pleasing behavior, and neither did I.

Several years later, I found myself in recovery describing the same traits. I had trouble saying "No." I tended to do what other people wanted to do. I let them choose the restaurant; I split whatever meals they wanted. I said sorry when it wasn't my fault and when there was nothing to apologize for.

I worried about what others thought of what I was wearing, my makeup, and sometimes even my haircut. I told them I liked that movie because they said they liked it. Oh, and I would also say, "I really like that band you like." I pretended to want the same things others wanted and to love the same things they loved. I tiptoed around anything that might upset them. Most of the time, I didn't do it consciously or even on purpose. I thought I was pleasing others, but it was all just selfishness.

You might still be asking yourself how this behavior could be selfish. It was selfish, because manipulating how I showed up in order to gain others' approval is indeed selfish. I was operating out of the delusion that anticipating others' judgments of me and then functioning so that I didn't run into them was selfless when it was not. My motive, conscious or otherwise, was seeking approval.

People-pleasing sounds like such a friendly phrase. People often describe themselves as people-pleasers because it sounds selfless. Although it is sometimes said in a self-deprecating way, and with a smirk, there is often this underlying implication that people-pleasers are good people. When someone says they are a people-pleaser, people sigh and say, "Oh, I know what that's like." It's almost as if the person wants pity and an award simultaneously. I say, let's try making us all stop each time and say, "I am an approval seeker." I bet we won't get the same sigh of agreement.

I recently read a post on Instagram that said, "Often people-pleasing has more to do with us wanting to be perceived as 'good' than actually pleasing other people." I would take it one step further and say it has nothing to do with pleasing other people and everything to do with selfishly seeking approval. There is no such thing as selflessly manipulating my own behavior to get the reaction that I desire out of you. People-pleasing behavior is always selfish, and it is routinely fear-based in my experience.

I was afraid of making my parents and teachers angry as a child and learned to avoid this by acting in certain ways. I made friends by showing up in certain ways and then developed fear of losing the friendships if I showed up any other way. I had had experiences of showing up authentically and then being rejected. I then held onto fear of future rejection, and that fear turned into people-pleasing behavior.

No matter the story I had for the behavior, the important piece was for me to sit down and see the fear and the selfish need for approval lurking below it all. It was the only way out of the fear, and the only path out of this behavior pattern. If you want to be truly loved by others and feel safe in relationships, showing up in dishonesty is not going to be the path to making that happen. I know from experience.

However, showing up constantly saying, "No," or behaving in a way that is aggressive, unkind, unloving, or unapologetic is also not the path out of people-pleasing behavior. I have used "No" as a full sentence in an unloving way and received in return the rejection that I deserved for the hurt I caused. Boundaries are not a panacea. My behavior has to be loving and God-centered, or it's actually a result of the need for approval's ugly and equally selfish cousin, resentment.

The path out of people-pleasing behavior was not to act like someone who isn't a people-pleaser. It was to see my behavior for what it was and bring it to God for help; only from that place could I begin to show up both lovingly and authentically. If you say something I don't agree with, something that scares me or challenges me, and I decide that continuing my personal path with God means I should stay quiet, that's amazing. It is not approval seeking because it is aligned with my best understanding of God's will for me at that moment. However, if I stay quiet because I am afraid of your reaction or that you won't like me if I disagree, then the problem is the selfish need for approval. I must be able to see these underlying motives in myself, one decision at a time.

What is most surprising is that my relationships are far better without approval seeking, "people-pleasing" behavior. People trust who I am when I show up. I am more forgiving; I am more loving. I don't expect things in return, not even approval. This was only made possible by understanding how selfish and self-centered my old behavior was. I prayed for relief from the need for approval and the underlying fears. I made sure to seek forgiveness for lingering anger about past instances of rejection and to forgive the individuals who had rejected me.

Today, I experience being far less sensitive to rejection and am, therefore, far more open to loving others without the strings of approval attached. I know that God's approval comes first, and people's approval comes last, or maybe even not at all. I know people love me for who I am, not because I want to do whatever they want to do. It's hard to say "No" to people. And without God by my side, I probably wouldn't be able to do it or would do it in unloving ways. But with God by my side, I just keep putting one foot in front of the other; His will always brings more peace and more love into my life, whether the answer to another human is "Yes" or "No."

Lesson 22

Dishonesty Runs Deeper Than I Realized

Without a relationship with God, there did not appear to be any consequences to dishonesty unless I hurt another human or broke a law. These consequences don't crop up nearly as often as dishonesty. And, when I did hurt another human being or break a law as a result of my own dishonesty, my tendency was to blame someone else for my feeling that I had to be dishonest, resent them for overreacting to my dishonesty, or deflect by breaking into tears and producing an apology that was not an apology for my dishonesty, but a plea to repair the relationship. Before I had a relationship with God, I had little sense of the need for truth, especially if I wasn't hurting anyone.

Before I knew God, my life was full of dishonesty. I am not here to say that everyone who has a distant or nonexistent relationship with God is dishonest, but I do believe that my distance from God did allow me to delve into deep levels of dishonesty, because, as I laid out earlier, there are few consequences when they are not viewed from a spiritual lens. For example, as a young adult, I regularly lied to my parents about where I was and who I was with in an effort to not get in trouble and control their beliefs about how I behaved. I can remember cheating on a spelling test in first grade—out of the fear that I would otherwise not get a good enough grade and let my parents down. I can remember cheating on boyfriends and lying about where I was and who I was with, fueled by fear that I needed a backup plan in case they broke up with me. If they never found out, who was I hurting?

There were other patterns of dishonesty that were a little less blatant that also started when I was young. I can remember my parents asking me if my chores were done, and that I told them, "Yes," but what I meant was that I would get them done. I said that assignments were nearly finished when they were barely started. I said that I listened to music that I had not listened to and said I had seen movies I had not seen with the intention of listening to the music or watching the movie in the future. I wanted to fit in, and who was I hurting?

It gets even more subtle. I wore fashionable clothes because I wanted people to believe certain things about me. I bought designer purses because people seemed to value and compliment people who had them. I made sure not to say things that might offend people because I wanted them to like me. I knew what to say to whom to appear to be a person that they would like. I was a social chameleon who could fit in with lots of different people and groups. The ability to read the room and act accordingly is seen as a character asset to many people, but is it? Is it not the ability to be subtly dishonest? Even if it is, who was I hurting?

Whether subtle or blatant, dishonesty appears whenever I manipulate or change anything about the truth in order to try to ensure a certain outcome. That is dishonesty, whether it happens in the form of a blatant lie, a purposeful omission, a subtle shift of the truth, or a hope that something will be true in the future if I just take action in time so that I can get away with pretending it's true now.

At the individual level, dishonesty was a sign that I was not willing to accept the consequences of my actions. I did not trust that the world would function in my best interest if I spoke and lived in the truth, so I lied.

At the interpersonal level, dishonesty is a signal that I am not in a relationship with a person I trust. If I cannot be honest with them, the relationship is already eroded. If I have to lie about how I spend my time, my energy, or my money, I am not actually in an intimate relationship, whether platonic or romantic. I am probably not fully loving them since I am in a perpetual state of dishonesty. And perhaps most importantly, I am certainly not allowing myself to be fully loved for who I am.

At the spiritual level, when I am dishonest, I am in essence sending a message to God that I do not trust Him with the outcome. If I feel the need to change the story, manipulate, or lie, I am saying to God that I do not trust the happenings that follow truth. I need to control it. I need to control what someone thinks—or what everyone thinks—in order to control how I feel.

When I am living in honesty and speaking truth, I am living from a place of trust, not just of myself or of others, but of God. So, who was my dishonesty hurting? Certainly others, at times. But, above all, I was hurting myself, because I was pushing myself further from God, further from faith, love, and truth. I was pushing myself further into distrust and disconnection. Dishonesty is always a sign that faith in God has eroded, and my honesty always indicates that I trust God with the outcome enough that I can tell the truth in all circumstances about who I am and what I am doing. This is because I trust that the outcome, whether it's what I wanted or not, is indeed what is best for me because it happened. When this happens, I move closer to intimacy not only with other humans, but also with my Creator. Some people call that moving toward Utopia, and it all starts with honesty.

Lesson 23

Guilt Is Not a Feeling

What if I told you that guilt is a fact, not a feeling, and that understanding this changed my life? I don't know when I was taught that guilt is a feeling, but that belief was one big misleading wild-goose chase into years of mind games and self-pity. I now understand the life-changing truth.

Guilt is not a feeling; guilt is a fact. Not only is guilt a fact, but when I accept my guilt, I am on the path to peace, and when I deny it, I am on the path to suffering.

Here's an example of how my life went when I thought guilt was a feeling. "I feel so guilty for cheating on him." So, I did feel super guilty. But then I remembered that he'd been a real jerk to me, and then I didn't feel so guilty. Until I remembered how thoughtful he was sometimes, and then I felt guilty again. After, I told one of my friends, and she told me that she would have cheated on him given everything that had been going on, and I felt less guilty again.

See how distorted my conscience becomes when I understand guilt as a feeling? I try to resolve the guilt with my thinking. And what are my options for getting through it? I have to rationalize my way out of it, hope other people are willing to tell me that I don't have to feel guilty, try to just forget about it, or perhaps just have a glass (or ten) of wine or take an edible to assist me in soothing it and forgetting about it, at least temporarily.

My life changed with the understanding that I don't *feel* guilty, I *am* guilty. I am guilty or I am not guilty. That's it. When I am not guilty, I feel peace. When I am guilty, I feel shame, remorse, and regret. Moreover, when I try to deny the guilt instead of facing it, I eventually end up in depression and despair on the one hand or anxiety and panic on the other, or perhaps a mix of the two. Historically, I tried to change these conditions with rationalization as well as alcohol, drugs, food, workouts, and the like without realizing that denied guilt was the root cause.

Let's say you are now convinced that guilt is a fact and that you realize that you are feeling the effects of denial of guilt, but now what? First, identify the guilt. Sometimes the guilt is obvious, as in this case. I am guilty of cheating on whomever this is. Other obvious candidates are if I am guilty of dishonesty or guilty of theft. It isn't so obvious all the time, however, that doesn't mean I am not guilty, it just means I need to dig a little deeper.

The examples are endless, but here are a few of the most common. When I am upset with someone for how they behaved, *I am usually guilty of judgment*. When the feeling of anger doesn't dissipate as quickly as it came, *I am usually guilty of resentment*. When I believe I was treated unfairly, *I am usually guilty of pride*. When I feel fearful, *I am usually guilty of self-centeredness or seeking self-centered goals*; the outcome I desire may not come to fruition. When I wish something about my life was different, *I am often guilty of envy*.

All right, guilty as charged; now what? I realize I am guilty, but what do I do with this newfound understanding? The real gift is that by accepting instead of denying that I am guilty and allowing God to enter my heart to forgive the guilt, I turn from a cheater into a *forgiven* cheater. I turn from a judge into a *forgiven* judge. I turn from a thief into a *forgiven* thief.

The acid test of whether I have truly allowed this forgiveness is not only whether I am at peace, but also whether I can love those who are guilty. When I am guilty, I have to separate from those who are guilty. "I can't believe she cheated on him!" will come out of my mouth. When I am *forgiven*, I instead have compassion for the guilty and am willing to share my past guilt with them in order to show them that when they are truly ready for forgiveness, it is always available to them, just as it was to me.

Forgiveness is always available, peace is always available, and the ability to effortlessly love others is always available. It requires me to stop denying my guilt and seek forgiveness. Until then, I get to stay separated from God and hold on to all the shame, remorse, and regret. But when I accept forgiveness, I have the capacity to love others, and I am at peace.

Lesson 24

Denial Takes Many Forms

Denial runs a lot deeper than I realized. Several months into my relationship with God, I was way too aware to be in denial. I had done the spiritual work—or so I thought. But as it turns out, I had only scratched the surface. For example, I was no longer in denial that I was a thief. I had previously tried to tell myself I wasn't a thief because I only shoplifted due to peer pressure, I was so young, and lots of teens go through that phase. But deep down, I always knew I was guilty. In the wee hours of the night, it had been on my mind. Through self-searching, I discovered and accepted that I was a thief. That was a good start, but I had buried most of my guilt a whole lot deeper, where it was barely on my mind at all.

For example, I actually convinced both myself and a past boyfriend that cheating on him was his fault because he had been emotionally distant, and besides, he had cheated on me first. I denied my guilt by rationalizing that he was also guilty. Was he wrong for cheating? Perhaps he was. But that is between him and his own conscience. More importantly, knowing whether he was wrong or not didn't change the fact that I was guilty.

Let's try an example of even deeper denial. When I was in fifth grade, a friend of mine was murdered, shot by his own mother; and for years, I was resentful and unforgiving of her. I believed I was completely justified in doing so. This one may be tough for some people to understand, but my awakening to the fact that I was guilty of resentment toward her and unforgiveness of her, and that it was harming me, not her, was a huge shift for me. Would society tell me that my resentment and unforgiveness were justified considering what she did? Absolutely yes. Was denying my guilt in this way still causing me pain? The answer is also absolutely yes, it was.

These are just three examples. Denial of guilt takes on many forms. One of the most perplexing aspects of denial is that we often bury the guilt so deeply that it becomes difficult to consciously access it at all. So, if you're wondering if you have denied guilt, here are some ways to quickly diagnose yourself. For me and others close to me, denial of guilt has manifested as anxiety disorders; despair and depression; angry outbursts; excessive exercise, drinking, drug use, gambling, or shopping; chronic physical pain; either obsessively working or changing jobs or projects often; moving often; not eating enough or overeating; controlling others or believing you know how others should behave; seeking new diagnoses from doctors or therapists; autoimmune conditions; pretending to be happy when you are not; and claiming that life would be happier if circumstances were different. The list could go on and on.

When I am exhibiting any of these behaviors or symptoms, it is usually because I am trapped in denial, and I tend to then react to that in two ways. First, I rationalize and justify my guilt: I was young, what they did was worse, I am only human, or you would do it, too, if you were in my position. I get myself, and sometimes also others, to believe that I am the victim. Second, I turn the focus toward the behaviors or symptoms of the denial of guilt instead of the guilt itself. For example, I have been injured from over-exercising, I have been diagnosed with eating disorders as well as anxiety and panic conditions, and I have been hospitalized for excessive drinking and drug use.

Those were never the real problem; my denial of my guilt was. However, those behaviors served as a perfect distraction from the real problem for me and for others. We all focused on the behaviors and diagnoses, blind to the reality that they resulted from my own feeble attempts to soothe the emotions that resulted from denied guilt.

These emotions began as shame, remorse, and regret. Over time, they developed into exhaustion and worry, eventually becoming depression and anxiety, and in the end, showed up as despair and panic. By denying my guilt, I was burning the candlestick at both ends, and I couldn't even see that it was my own denial that had brought me to that point.

The first step out of this painful blindness was surrendering to the fact that these behaviors, symptoms, rationalizations, justifications, and emotions were signs of denied guilt. I was on the road to the solution when I recognized that denial of guilt was certainly my primary problem, if not my only problem. The next step was finding the guilt I was denying. Using the three examples I began with above, I stole, I cheated, and I was resentful and unforgiving. When I was able to accept that I was indeed guilty, I took this previously denied guilt to the Divine Physician for forgiveness and healing.

What that looks like for me is saying, "God, I was wrong. I was in total denial, but now I can see." When that prayer comes not only from my mind, but also from my heart, peace enters. Sometimes it looks peaceful, and sometimes I burp, weep, or even shake. Nevertheless, I know that the guilt is finally released, and I experience the unconditional love of divine forgiveness, sometimes also referred to as grace. Turning to God with that prayer was the foundation of my recovery from all the behaviors and symptoms associated with my denied guilt and remains the foundation of my ever-continuing path to more consistent peace of soul.

Lesson 25

The Paradox of Insecurity

One morning last summer, as I was getting ready to go wakesurfing with a group of friends, I suddenly laughed to myself as I realized that I had worn the same swimsuit every time for the entire summer. That swimsuit was the one on the top of the swimsuit bin, and I just kept picking it back up. This may seem minor, but I used to absolutely obsess about what I was going to wear to any given event. How does this swimsuit look on this particular day? Is this the right outfit? I would change many, many times. That day, I put a swimsuit on without even looking in the mirror and hopped on my motorcycle to head to the lake. In fact, these days, I am now sometimes caught off guard when someone says, "I love your outfit," because I have forgotten what I was wearing. In the past, I would have done anything for a compliment like that.

I also remember that just a couple years ago, I was painfully nervous about what I was going to talk to people about at events. I did not know what questions to ask. What if I talked about the wrong thing and I seemed weird? What if it was not the cool thing to talk about? What if someone adamantly disagreed with what I was saying?

I could not even decide what I wanted to do or eat because I wanted to make sure that everyone else was happy with it. I unknowingly made a variety of situations confusing for others. I wasn't hungry unless they were. I did not want to go to the fair or get on that ride unless they did. I didn't even want to change seats at the movie theater unless my companions could confirm that they agreed the other seats were better.

I also read way too far into other people's decisions. For example, on another night last summer, a couple of friends came over to help with some last-minute tasks related to my wedding. I offered to buy them dinner when we were done, and they both declined. In the past, I would have wondered if I had done or said something wrong, or if I had made them work too hard and they were annoyed with me. Yesterday, however, I just said "okay," and they went home.

I have found that one of the pieces of the puzzle underlying a lot of the anxiety I have felt in life is "what others think of me," whether what they thought of me was real or imagined. What do I mean by real or imagined? Sometimes, it was the true opinion of others that I was worried about. Perhaps I know that my friend Janet cares a lot about appearance and judges people based on it. Perhaps, sometimes it was imagined, just a general nervousness about what others thought of me or a discomfort with "being myself," a sense of discomfort that left me anxious and changing my outfit five times before I left the house.

If you can identify with any of these feelings, then you might be suffering from the oppression of concern with what others think of you, just as I used to (and on rare occasions, still do). What's worse, like me, you might think that the only solution is to just *try* not to care while still quietly suffering or simply doing your best to suppress the suffering.

What if I told you there is another way? That way is understanding that the suffering is all within you, that it is all various forms of the need for approval. I wasn't pleasing others; I was seeking approval for myself. I was anxiously avoiding losing others' approval, and I was doing it so often that I wasn't even aware that I was doing it. The first step was realizing just how often I was doing it.

Next came prayer. Each and every time that I became aware that I was thinking about or nervous about what someone else was thinking, I would pray for God's help, for relief from the need for approval.

Moreover, if there was a pattern, I asked for help to see that pattern. For example, I had an old belief that I had to look a certain way in a swimsuit. This was an old belief that was conditioned into me that took the form of resentment. In other words, I watched someone get made fun of for how their swimsuit looked and then was desperately trying to avoid the same fate for myself in a subconscious way. The way out was to not only pray for relief from my fear of being ridiculed, but also, more importantly, to pray for forgiveness for my resentment toward the original swimsuit bully. My anger toward her was the root of all the associated fear. You are never so fearful as when you are angry. Moreover, throughout my life, I was guilty of judging others for how they looked, and that guilt was also rearing its head in the form of my own insecurity. Once I was forgiven of the judgment, the insecurity fell away, too.

The bottom line is that I needed to realize that there is always resentment or fear underlying any thought concerning what another person thinks of me. The way out is not to tell myself not to care what they think, it is to pray for God's help for release from the underlying resentment and fear. Over time, when I did that consistently, I came out the other side free. By free, I mean I no longer have to try to figure out how not to care what others think, it just doesn't come to mind.

Lesson 26

There Is a Solution to Anxiety

I recently took a call from a friend who was starting to date someone new. She was feeling anxious. Her worries ranged from minor concerns, such as when this man was going to text her back, to larger concerns, such as whether he really liked her, whether he was talking to other women, and whether she should even be dating at all.

The conversation took me back to what my dating life was like before I had a relationship with God. I was full of very similar anxieties and fears. They were not necessarily based on any behavior that the man I was dating at any given time had displayed. He could be completely attentive and answer texts and calls in a reasonable amount of time, yet I would still find I was full of anxiety. In fact, at the time I met my husband, I did not have the relationship with God I have today, and I distinctly remember having these kinds of anxieties about him.

Friends told me that this kind of anxiety was normal and that everyone experiences some jitters early in a relationship. Although I appreciated my friends trying to make me feel normal, I knew that my anxiety level was not normal. Moreover, I now see normalizing anxiety as simply normalizing an unnecessary experience of suffering. Just because an experience is common does not mean that it is one that is necessary.

So, if the experience, while common, is not necessary, how does one avoid it? For me, I first had to understand that my present experience of anxiety was being caused by past anger. Let me share an example of this. Early on when my husband, Kevin, and I were dating, I saw an email pop up on his phone that was from a woman. I immediately spiraled into anxiety that he was cheating on me, even though my anxiety had nothing to do with the present situation. I was anxious because seeing the email had triggered a boatload of past anger.

It had triggered anger that I was holding onto about men who would talk to me and other women at the same time and men who had cheated on me while we were dating. It had also triggered old anger I had not dealt with related to rejection I experienced in relationships with boys as early as elementary school.

This mountain of past anger was the catalyst for my anxiety about the email my husband received; so the only way to get rid of the anxiety was to get rid of the past anger. Therefore, I not only went to work on forgiving each of the men, but I also took my anger toward them to God for healing. I prayed to God for relief from my anger toward each and every one of them, as well as for help in forgiving any past harms. I did this again and again until I felt that I had truly worked through the anger.

Then something beautiful happened. I was no longer carrying my past into the present. I was no longer showing up full of trigger buttons; therefore, I was no longer triggered. I can't even remember what happened with the email, but I don't think I even cared about it after I had worked through my past anger. I could see that my anxiety had not been related to Kevin at all; it was simply a symptom of all of my past anger.

The beautiful thing is that doing the work doesn't just relieve the anxiety of a single situation, it allows me to continue to live in the present without carrying the weight of my past with me. Today, I have zero fear that Kevin is secretly emailing other women. Can I say with

100 percent certainty that he is not? Well, no. But I can say with 100 percent certainty that I don't have anxiety about it. That doesn't mean I don't trust my husband; I truly don't think he is in a secret relationship. The point is not whether his behavior is perfect, rather the point is that I live in serenity whether it is or not.

Although this example has been about relationships, this spiritual principle that anxiety is often just a symptom of anger is not unique to relationships. My money anxiety was related to anger I had about finances, including my own finances, general financial inequality, and even jealousy of others' finances. My anxiety about body image was deeply connected to anger I had about my body and other people's bodies. My anxiety about the health and welfare of my family was related to anger I had about what I perceived to be untimely and unfair illnesses and death. My social anxiety was directly tied to anger I had about being left out and misunderstood as a child. I truly believe my generalized anxiety was just a symptom of the mountain of anger I had across the board. Why do I believe that? Since offering others and the world unconditional forgiveness and going to God for forgiveness from my own anger, I have seen a dramatic decrease in my anxiety. And on the flip side, when anger pops up, anxiety often comes back with it.

It was hard to admit that I was deeply angry. Anxiety is a much nicer word and a much more socially acceptable state of suffering. Nevertheless, to admit I was angry and allow God to heal my anger was the end of my anxious suffering. I encourage you to at least ask yourself if your life would be better without anxiety. If so, maybe it's time to take a look at your anger. Doing so changed my life.

Lesson 27

There Is a Way Out of the Cycle of Shame

Has anyone ever said something negative to you that stuck with you for years? Maybe someone told you that you wouldn't amount to anything—that you were too fat, thin, tall, or short, or that you weren't smart enough or pretty enough. Perhaps you just have been telling yourself these things for ages even though you can't pinpoint anyone ever having said them to you.

Many scholars have written about the nature of shame. What they tend to agree on is that it boils down to pain caused by an internalization of being unlovable. It is a deeply held belief that "I am not enough."

I recently heard someone telling a story about shame that I hope will be useful because of its simplicity. A man in his fifties said that when he was a child, a girl walked up to him and told him that he was the second ugliest boy in the whole school. He said that to this day, every time he gets dressed and looks in the mirror, he can still hear what she said—and he still feels shame remembering her words.

I, too, used to suffer from a lot of shame. I remembered moments when people commented on my body and other people's bodies, and the result was that I felt body shame. I heard others talking about how close their friendships were, and I felt shame that I didn't have closer friends. People made comments about my clothes, and I felt ashamed that I didn't have money for trendier clothes. People told me they didn't like my boyfriend, and I became ashamed of my relationship.

Sometimes I would try to talk myself out of some of these with logical arguments, but it never really worked. Deep down I had a sense of being not enough.

But the question remains, what is shame? I treated shame as if it was something for which people should pity me because it resulted from negative things others said to me or that I experienced. The consequence of believing this was that I was just digging myself deeper into what the real problem was. The real difficulty and the root of the shame were not what someone said to me, what happened to me, or what someone else did to me. It was my resentment, leading to my guilt for being resentful. Remember, guilt is not a feeling, guilt is a fact.

I will try to explain by taking you back to the first example. The man had an experience in which a girl called him ugly, and that led him to truly believe that he was ugly, which he then experienced as shame.

The root of the problem is not what the girl said to him. That happened, but it's been over for years. The root of his shame is his unforgiven resentment toward the girl. He is in the pain of shame because of his resentment toward her. If he goes to God for forgiveness for this resentment and then forgives the girl, the shame will fade away. If he stays in resentment, he will keep the shame.

If you are surprised that the problem is within you, don't worry, I was surprised to find out the problem was within me. However, when I could get past my surprise and find the core of my resentment, and then bring that to God, the shame disappeared. When I chose to stay in resentment, I stayed ashamed. When I tried to forgive with my head and not my heart, I was still ashamed following the attempt. When I felt any negative feelings toward a person, society, or anything else I blamed, I found that I was not done with the resentment and that I remained ashamed. When I instead saw my resentment as the problem, brought that to God, and finally let go, the shame faded away.

Sometimes shame results from a specific resentment connected to a specific person or situation, such as the ones described above. Sometimes, it is more general. For example, I was convinced that the Victoria's Secret Angels and society's standards of beauty were causing me to have body shame. But they were not causing my body shame. It was my resentment of their existence that was causing me shame. When I prayed about my resentment toward Victoria's Secret Angels as well as general societal standards of beauty, my body shame began to fade.

One of the most insidious aspects of shame for me was that I was convinced that it was an unavoidable aspect of life. I thought that it was the result of the things that had happened to me—which couldn't be further from the truth. The truth is that shame is completely avoidable, and that it is a direct result of me being in a state of resentment and unforgiveness. Since I am the one in denial, the truth is that I am the one who needs forgiveness. If I am unwilling to go to God for forgiveness or unwilling to forgive whomever I believe hurt me, then the shame will continue.

However, when those two pieces are dealt with, my experience is that 100 percent of the time, the shame is gone. Dealing with shame is an ongoing process because new hurts will happen. But when I am willing to take responsibility for my shame on a continual basis, it means that no matter what happens to me, I know that I will not be sitting around suffering from shame. I was always enough and always lovable, and what was blocking me from that knowledge wasn't other people, society, or my past, it was my own resentment and unforgiveness blocking me from experiencing freedom.

Lesson 28

Alcoholics Are Hard on Holidays

A common phrase I have heard from many therapists is, "Holidays are hard on alcoholics," relating to helping clients to soothe their fears about heading home for the holidays. And it is true that for an active alcoholic or addict, holidays are almost invariably messy. When I was in active addiction, I was usually hung over from drinking or overeating. I was often focused more on what I was going to eat or drink next than on enjoying conversation with my family or friends. I was irritable; I was discontent; I was anxious. I was easily triggered by difficult topics of discussion. When things didn't go as planned or even simply as I expected, I was all the more irritable. Holidays were always a reminder that my parents were divorced, and that my family was not a Hallmark family. This was not because there was anything inherently wrong with my family's structure or the structure of any family, but because I was deeply enmeshed in my own victimhood.

To be clear, these character traits were not a direct result of drinking, using, or overeating. They are common among all kinds of individuals separated from God. I spent my first sober Thanksgiving separate from my family. And oh, the self-centered stories I had about not being with my family that day. And boy, did I use that story to garner pity from others. Again, although it was unconscious at the time, I was just too caught up in my own story to realize I was in a relentless cycle of victimhood.

Whether I was drinking or not, one of the most difficult aspects of my being an addict who was yet to find deep recovery in a relationship with

God was that I was extremely selfish and hard to be around. What's worse is that I had no idea that I was a difficult person at that point. I would have sworn that everyone else was hard to be around. I wished people would not make it necessary for *me* to have to walk on eggshells. They either cared too much about what I had been doing that day or the night before, or they were not interested enough in me and my life. It was worse when I was left out completely.

As an unrecovered addict, I had certain personality characteristics that were quite common. I was very selfish, in that I spent most of my time thinking about myself, whether in pride, pity, or obsession about what others thought of me. I didn't really care about other people as I should have because I was too lost in myself. And yes, serving others because I wanted them to like me was equally self-centered. Most of the time, I did not see my faults when conflicts arose. I primarily saw and ruminated on others' faults in each situation. I would show up to a holiday event and metaphorically step on other people's toes. When they retaliated, I would blame them for causing the holiday disturbance. "Hey, what are you doing that for? I didn't do anything to you." Except, I did; I did do something to that person, even though it might have been as simple as moping around the house in my self-pity or trying to control and change others because of my anxiety. I was just not aware of my behavior.

I was a bull in a China shop who thought I was a butterfly. I was not landing softly at holiday events. I was not bringing wonder and joy. I was barreling through, hoping to get what I wanted without realizing the wreckage that I was leaving in the wake of my unconscious self-centeredness because I couldn't even see that I was doing it. I only did what I wanted to do—events and activities that made me feel good. Pop psychology told me that was the nature of boundaries. And, maybe it is, but it is not the nature of the path to love, surrender, and peace.

The people I liked most were those I could control, or who happened to do what I wanted and expected. The people I felt were causing the most harm in my life were people who didn't live up to one or both of those criteria. I would say, "You are making me feel this way, and my feelings are valid." They would retort, "You are making me feel this way, and my feelings are valid." The only thing valid about our feelings is that we were both validating that we were allowed to retain our anger toward one another and express it as "having emotions," rather than taking the anger to God for forgiveness and truly loving each other.

The essential problem across all these behaviors was that I used the delusional story I told myself about my life to excuse my behavior. Meanwhile, I was inflicting self-harm and harm to others, and damaging my relationship with God. If the problem wasn't me, then there wouldn't have been a solution. Luckily, the problem was me, and it was, first and foremost, my inability to clearly see myself, my behavior, and my complete separation from God. The good news is that I did find a solution—namely, awareness of the truth about myself, understanding that I was in a lot more trouble than I thought I was, and that what I needed was reconciliation with God.

When I did this, the holidays became very different because I no longer focused on myself. I now have no expectations. I show up as God would have me show up. If I experience a negative feeling, I know it's a form of resentment, and that the resentment is in me, not anyone else. It is no one's fault but mine, and taking it to God is the only solution. I am neither anxious nor walking on eggshells. I am no longer triggered by difficult discussion topics or perspectives that aren't the same as my own. I am not disturbed by others' behavior. Plans can change without my mood changing. I know the structure of my family is exactly what it is supposed to be, and each family member's personality is as it should be and not meant for me to change.

I now realize that I used to have a bunch of feelings and ideas about how the holidays should go, grounded firmly in the lies I was telling myself. I realize that holidays are not hard on alcoholics, alcoholics are hard on holidays. I realize that the holidays have never been hard on me, it was always that I was hard on the holidays. And today, I am easy on the holidays and the holidays are easy on me, and the grace of God is to thank for that.

Lesson 29

Understanding the Pain of Uncertainty

Do you remember being in school and taking exams? As I think back on my days of taking tests, two situations stick out to me as being the most emotionally difficult. First and foremost, there was the anticipation of what questions would be on the test, along with the dread that I was potentially totally wasting my time studying content that wouldn't be on it. Second, the waiting period between taking the exam and getting my grade back was also very emotionally difficult.

What they have in common is the experience of uncertainty. The questions were completely out of my control, yet I still felt compelled to prepare for the test to the best of my ability. So, I put all kinds of time and effort into an uncertain outcome. The second situation was difficult because there was nothing I could do but wait.

Here's what I know for sure. In college, uncertainty was a painful experience. And even today, it is still sometimes that way. I can't count the number of times I have said something along the lines of, "If it's bad news, that's okay, I would just prefer to know." I know this was true for the RSVPs for my wedding last year. Getting RSVPs back that were a "No" was no problem. It was the people who didn't respond that put me on an emotional roller coaster.

So, why does uncertainty fill me with so much anxiety? Unfortunately, the diagnosis appears to be because it is simply triggering my need for control. High need for control leads to high levels of pain in the face of uncertainty. Low need for control means lower pain in the face of uncertainty. When I have no need for control, I experience no pain in the face of uncertainty. And what's the real diagnosis of the need for control?

Lack of faith.

The real problem is my faith. Underneath my anxiety is a belief that if I can just keep everything and everyone in place, I will be okay. It's a total lack of acknowledgement that God has everything covered. It's rarely a conscious dismissal of my faith. I don't declare that I need control and don't trust God. My pain is just a sign that my faith is on shaky ground.

I know this to be true, because here's what is fascinating. When my faith is strong, uncertainty does not feel painful. There is no emotional roller coaster or anxious tailspin. I have not taken a test in the last few years, so I can't speak for how my faith would work in relation to an exam today, but I can describe how it has changed a lot of other situations.

The future of my career is currently uncertain. When I finally handed it to God, it stopped even coming up in my mind. Whether I will ever get pregnant is something only God knows, and it is a question that I was struggling with for several months before I truly turned it over to God. Now it rarely bothers me, and when it does, I turn back to prayer. My husband is quite a bit older than me, and I used to have anxiety about what my life would look like if I married him because chances are I'll outlive him by thirty or forty years. I finally turned it over to God, and I trust that whatever happens is exactly what is supposed to happen. Despite my tenuous job situation, we are looking for a house, and the uncertainty surrounding finding and financing a house is something that I know I would not be able to handle without a loving God to whom I can give my problems.

God gives me the serenity to accept the things I cannot change and the wisdom to know what those things are. It is not something that I can think my way out of; I have to pray my way out of it. In fact, telling myself, "Don't worry about it, Lisa. You don't have control over it." leads to no more serenity than worrying about it because *thinking is not praying.*

Trying to think myself into not experiencing the pain of uncertainty is not the same as praying to God to relieve the pain and replace it with faith. The former is intellectualizing my problem, the latter is putting my trust in the Creator of the Universe that His plan, which happens to dissolve pain, is better than my plan. Today, when I get caught up in the pain of uncertainty, I don't chastise myself or try to think my way out of it. Instead, I recognize it, hit my knees, and tell God that I trust His plan completely.

PART III

Debunking Self-Help and Trendy Spirituality

Lesson 30

Trusting God Isn't Trendy

I always had this aching internal sense that there was more to life than what I knew. Over time, my explorations led me to the conclusion that spirituality was the answer, but, oh my, was it complicated. I followed podcasts and blogs created by people who claimed to be starseeds and celestial beings. I had tarot cards. I knew my human design. I knew my astrology and numerology. I had all sorts of crystals. I knew the difference between a plant shaman and a spirit shaman. I knew that if I sent negative vibes to a glass of water, upon freezing, it would crystallize differently than if I sent kindness to it. I had taken a training course to be a psychic medium. I had books on being witchy and on channeling spirits. I was a two-hundred-hour certified yoga instructor in power yoga, which is perhaps one of the less "spiritual" yoga traditions, but I had also dabbled in kundalini yoga as well as breathwork and sound healing. I had done meditations on past lives and reparenting my inner child, both assisted and not assisted by psychedelics.

I was also deeply embedded in the connection between wellness trends and spirituality; I was always trying to raise my vibration with the next wellness solution, ranging from raw food to keto to red lights, infrared saunas, colon hydrotherapy, cryotherapy, ice baths, beds of nails, acupuncture, and herbalism. If I could stay aligned with my intentions and gratitude, I believed my desires would manifest, and that this was indeed how the universe was supposed to work. This was the secret.

The thing that all these behaviors and beliefs have in common is that among my trendy, highly educated, urban-dwelling peers, these didn't ruffle any feathers and, in fact, made me seem more intelligent and awakened. After all, my PhD in psychology proved I knew better than to believe that "regular old God" as I called it—the biblical God—was a thing, let alone *the* thing.

The people around me, albeit mostly not particularly serene individuals, tended toward this brand of spirituality as well. They didn't want people thinking they were judgmental, hypocritical, or simple-minded, and they thought God-people were. If I chose my own personal brand of spirituality, I could avoid contending with these prejudices. So, the best route was nontraditional spirituality. For me, this was the universe, the spirit that connects us all—nature and the energy that flows everywhere.

My true awakening began when I realized that at bottom, even with the universe on my side, I still wasn't at peace. Something deep down inside me told me that there was more to life, and the truth was that the uneasy, uncomfortable, aching feeling that was always within me had never fully dissipated. Eventually, this internal ache escalated to the point that I was willing to be open, to drop my prejudices against believers and my fear of judgment from nonbelievers, and to try anything, and finally that included God, Creator of the Universe—not the universe, the creator.

I didn't understand God that first day, and I don't today. I think that's the way it's supposed to be. But I chose faith, the mystery of faith, and lo and behold, my life changed. I finally began to experience an inner peace like nothing I had experienced before, and I began to trust God, not the universe or new age spirituality, trendy and easy on the ears of the over-educated, just God, regular old God. And not just belief in God, but faith.

Here is the truth: I don't have all the answers, and I know that trusting God isn't trendy.

If you're doing headstands with crystals, I am not saying that's wrong. I can't and don't want to make that call. I also do know that there are some benefits to many of the practices I tried, but I also know that these do not work for me, and often even work against me, when I use them apart from God. When I bring God with me, He shows me which ones to move toward and which ones are not for me.

I also know that new age manifestation no longer made sense once I had faith. The best possible outcome, partner, house, or day is the one that God has in store for me, and it is so much greater than anything I could come up with on my own. Not greater in the material sense, but greater in that they are each exactly what they are supposed to be. That is the real secret. It's not manifesting what I want, it's finding God, letting go of what I think I want, and finding something much greater.

Lesson 31

I Was Searching for Spirituality in All the Wrong Places

A few days ago, I was sitting with some friends, and one asked whether the feeling of God is any different than the feelings that I found when I was in the world of drugs, alcohol, and non-God "spirituality." She had never experienced the feeling of being on mushrooms or MDMA, having her tarot cards read, or channeling beings from other planets. I am not sure she had ever even experienced regular old drunkenness the way I had either. But the question is still important. Is there a difference?

The reason why I did all of those things was because I was seeking to feel something different. I was seeking out these worldly things because I was looking for communion with others, fun, joy, peace, and a sense of being at home in the world. At the time, I am not sure that I could even fully explain what I was searching for nor even that I was suffering because I had stuffed my pain down so well for so many years and was deeply dissociated from much of it. I had gotten so used to being in pain that I didn't really realize the amount of pain I was in. I knew that I felt anxious, I knew I had stomach problems, I knew I wasn't comfortable in my own skin. I knew that I just wanted to feel happy and a part of something.

And here is the weird part. Psychedelics, tarot, self-focused meditation, channeling, and the like actually worked pretty well as a respite. I call them *sensate pleasures*. If the feeling of doing those things was not pleasurable, people wouldn't do them, and they certainly wouldn't get lost in them. I was lost in them. I thought that the sensation of pleasure was a spiritual awakening. I wasn't awakening, however, I was actually falling further asleep, even though I certainly didn't see it that way.

This happens with behaviors that aren't so dramatic as well. Even something as simple as a yoga class or a self-help book can produce such a respite. Each experience produced a shot of the delusion that I had found the answer to life and to remaining at peace. I know that effect well. On paper, I am a certified yoga instructor, and I have purchased and now donated more self-help books than I could ever count. In fact, looking back, I didn't even have to open the self-help book. I felt better just having it, walking out through the parking lot of the bookstore.

What I have started to experience over the last three years is something very different than the sensate pleasures of these drugs and "spiritual" practices. I have experienced a relationship with God. The feeling is in some ways much like the feelings I experienced during some of these past activities, but the energy of it is cleaner.

There is no desperation. There is no acting. There is no song and dance. There is no proving anything. There is no right position to stand in or sit in. There is no right outfit. There is no ingestion of any substance needed.

My Higher Power met me right where I was and filled my heart with the true spirit of God. And it felt different. The love was bigger and bolder, and it positively changed me so much faster than any of those other practices. The change was sudden and profound. I can't even remember my old way of thinking and feeling. And it just keeps getting better and better.

There is no guru. There is no one to pay. There are no drugs I need to take. There are no specific ceremonies. There is just me and God. Interestingly, the quieter I get and the more I empty myself, the stronger the feeling of God is. The pomp of the other ceremonies in my previous pursuits was a sensate pleasure. With God, it is just being in His presence that changes me. The rest, oddly enough, comes just by spending time with Him.

But what about praying? I can guarantee you that if you spend time with God, you will want to pray. What about confession of wrongs? Once again, I never feel more aware of my own patterns and defects nor any stronger conviction about how God's love can change them than after I spend time with God.

The life I had always been searching for, a life filled with communion with others, fun, joy, peace, and a sense of being at home in the world, came to me through my relationship with God, and it is available to everyone. It doesn't take a flight to Costa Rica. It doesn't take someone explaining what love is. The feeling of God is love because God is love. It is nothing like any ceremony you have ever tried. If you love the ceremonies and I can't convince you otherwise, no problem. Keep doing them until you reach the end of the road like I did. Only at the end of the road was I open-minded enough to see and to seek the God who created all the ceremonies. So, participate in all the ceremonies you like. God won't leave your side, and He will be ready when you are.

Lesson 32

The Problem with Gratitude Lists

Take out a piece of paper. Write a gratitude list, one with just three things on it. Here's mine. "I am grateful for the roof over my head. I am grateful for this warm cup of coffee with steamed soy milk that my husband brought to me in bed. I am grateful for my relationship with my mother."

Great job! Do you feel a little lighter? Perfect. Let's hope it lasts through the full lesson.

We just engaged in the practice of something I have come to call *artificial gratitude*. Artificial gratitude is gratitude that I purposefully choose to engage in, gratitude that comes out of my intellect. This type of gratitude is popular. People everywhere seem to think life would be better if they could just remember to make their gratitude list or fill up their gratitude journal. Or perhaps, like me, you were making your lists and filling up your journals, and you couldn't understand why you weren't feeling much better.

I must imagine that the original idea for gratitude lists developed from someone's good intentions, perhaps something like, "Scientists studied the happiest people on Earth, those with the most contentment, and found that they have gratitude." The answer, so they think, is to consciously produce more gratitude. But what if that isn't the answer? I had to ask myself, how were my gratitude lists going?

Was I living life in a constant or even mostly constant state of contentment? Short answer: No.

My experience is that artificial gratitude is like a fast-acting aspirin: it's a great short-term solution that doesn't treat the root of the problem. I get to feel like I am doing something rather than nothing about my otherwise less than contented state, I get a feel-good feeling fast, and I get to say that I am the kind of person who writes gratitude lists regularly. However, the contentment I felt was always temporary, minutes or maybe hours at most. Metaphorically speaking, taking another aspirin never got to the root cause of the headache, and after a while, it wasn't even working all that well to relieve the pain.

So, if the answer to having more gratitude wasn't more gratitude lists, what was it? Ironically, instead of making gratitude lists, I started doing the opposite. I started making ungrateful lists. What was I not grateful for? What was blocking me from gratitude? What upset me? What was I worried about? For example, looking back at my first gratitude list, although I am grateful that I have a roof over my head, maybe I am frustrated that the roof over my head isn't in a better neighborhood.

Okay, so I am not grateful after all, now what? I find that trying to find gratitude for the roof I have over my head despite my frustration isn't nearly as effective at producing long-term contentment as getting to the bottom of the frustration lurking in my heart. So, ungrateful list in hand, I sit down and find the root of the problem, which starts with prayer for help finding the root issue. When I remain open to the answer, it always comes, not always right away, but it comes.

For example, maybe I find that I fear I will never move into a neighborhood where I feel safe or where I can raise kids the way I believe they should be raised. Perhaps I just selfishly wish that I could get more approval from others by having a better house to show off or to host gatherings. Maybe I am frustrated because I could afford a better home if I hadn't spent money so recklessly in the past or dated that guy with the spending problem. What I inevitably find is that whenever I am not grateful, I am living in some form of self-centeredness. Admitting this is tough, but when I can get there, everything changes.

That is because when I have the facts about myself in hand, I turn to God, admit my wrong, and accept the lasting relief that has always been available to me. No more temporary relief from artificial gratitude. This lasting relief comes in the form of forgiveness for my selfishness in whatever form it took (e.g. anger, jealousy, or fear). The result is that I end up lighter, in a stable state of contentment, and full of *organic gratitude*, gratitude that emanates from my heart as a result of freedom from any lurking heaviness, not gratitude that I've manufactured in my head to cover up the heaviness. In other words, my experience is that it is the absence of ungratefulness that leads to contentment and the presence of organic gratitude, not the addition of artificial gratitude confetti to an ongoing pity party.

So, for me, the cause of true contentment has not been to create more artificial gratitude. Instead, I turn to self-examination and prayer and find release from what I am not grateful for. The result is an abundance of organic gratitude and stable contentment. This method is simple, but not easy, and it may perhaps be counterintuitive, but all the best lessons are.

Lesson 33

How to Stop Negative Self-Talk

When I was fifteen years old, I started going to therapy for my eating disorder. Over the next fourteen years, I went to several therapists for issues ranging from various forms of eating disorders to anxiety, depression, and substance abuse. Here is an example of what happens in these sessions. I say, "I just hate myself; I don't understand why I can't get my eating disorder under control. I am never going to be able to recover. All my friends hate me, and I am making them miserable. I know my friend told me I am doing better, but she just said that to be nice. I should be able to just get through this." The therapist says something like, "Let's focus on some cognitive distortions and negative thought patterns you expressed here and try to reframe them. Then I want you to practice doing this throughout the week."

So, let's identify just a few thought patterns I had in my example conversation. First, when I said I would never be able to get my eating disorder under control or recover, I expressed some all-or-nothing thinking, also known as black-and-white thinking. I could have reframed that thought by realizing that I had experienced periods of time in the past when I was doing better; therefore, I was most likely not, in fact, doomed forever.

Then I engaged in overgeneralization when I said that all my friends hated me, as well as personalization when I assumed that the misery my friends experienced was about me. I could have reframed those thoughts and realized that it's certainly not all my friends who hate me. Not to mention that they are also going through their own stuff that has nothing to do with me, which might have been causing them some misery.

I then engaged in disqualifying the positive when I assumed my friend had just complimented me to be nice rather than because she actually believed it. I could have instead chosen to believe that she meant the compliment and accepted that maybe I was doing better. Finally, I used a "should" statement. Maybe I could have instead realized that I was making progress just by showing up to therapy instead of focusing on what I should be doing.

Each of these thought patterns is identified by psychological science as a cognitive distortion, and I had engaged in five of them: all-or-nothing thinking, overgeneralization, personalization, disqualifying the positive, and a "should" statement. Therapists would tell me that I just needed to practice, practice, practice at recognizing these and reframing the thoughts and all will be well. Fourteen years into therapy, I could understand that I needed to reframe the thoughts, and I had been doing it. I had journaled about my thinking, meditated on it, and talked to others about it. I had come to understand on an intellectual level that these were all just cognitive distortions and not reality. But I was still having them. Nothing was really changing.

To me, trying to change my thinking with my thinking was like writing a new thought on top of an old one on a chalkboard without erasing the original thought, not just once but for a lifetime. So, there wasn't just one negative thought along with a reframed thought on the chalkboard, there was a lifetime of thoughts and the thoughts with which I had tried to override them written on the chalkboard. Eventually, I couldn't read any of them, and I felt more confused than ever. When I tried to change my thinking with my thinking, I ended up feeling like a chalkboard full of gibberish and a jumbled mess.

In a recovery book that I read frequently, there is a line that says, "He finally realizes that he has undergone a profound alteration in his reaction to life; that such a change could hardly have been brought about by himself alone. What often takes place in a few months could seldom have been brought about by years of self-discipline." After fourteen years of self-discipline assisted by science and therapy, I was ready to try something different to change my thinking, that is, my reaction to life. I found that what I had tried to accomplish for years with self-discipline suddenly took place in a matter of months. I indeed had a profound alteration in my reaction to life.

This alteration in my thinking was not brought about by new ways of thinking nor by reframing my thoughts; as the book states, it was not brought about by me alone. It was brought about by prayer, more specifically, prayers of confession of my wrongs. Therapy had given me fancy intellectual words like cognitive distortion when all I was really doing was denying my guilt. Recognizing the selfishness, self-centeredness, fear, judgment, anger, and the like underneath each thought and going to God for forgiveness turned out to be the solution. I had to be honest with myself. I was not a victim of my thoughts, I was just a selfish, angry, fearful person.

As I took each thought to God, He slowly but surely erased each of the thoughts on the chalkboard of my mind. Slowly but surely, my mind became a blank slate. It isn't filled with negative thoughts. It also isn't filled with reframed thoughts nor positive affirmations. It is just sitting open and ready for new experiences and inspiration. So, if you're stuck in negative thinking, turning it over to God might just be worth a try.

Lesson 34

Self-Love Is Not What I Thought It Was

Self-love is not what I thought it was. In fact, I want nothing to do with it.

I thought I didn't love myself. I was self-conscious. I had the ability to be in a room with my friends and still feel like I didn't quite belong. I always wished my body was a different shape or size. I wished I had closer friendships. I wished I had more money. I wished my family was closer or less discombobulated. I chose boyfriends expecting that I would feel better about myself in the gleam of their love, but that never quite worked. I did well in school and in sports. I had a lot to be proud of. It just never quite made an impact. The solution, I believed, was to go on a self-love journey.

There were the early stages of trying to understand self-love. For me, these consisted of goals I should try to fulfill to achieve self-esteem. If I just lose these five pounds or drink that much green juice, then I will love myself. If I just save the money for this or that, then I will love myself. It was important that I keep promises to myself because I was told it builds self-trust and self-love. It is so clear to me now that I was way off the mark, but I couldn't see it at the time.

Then there was the next level of the self-love journey, during which I realized that it isn't about loving myself when I reach X, Y, or Z goal, but loving myself right now, just as I am. When I failed, love myself. No matter my body weight, love myself. No matter what clothing I can afford, love myself. No matter whether I am single or partnered, love myself. No matter where I live, love myself. Prove to the world that I not only exist, but that I am above the material world and can love myself in any and all circumstances. I don't even need the things other people need; I just need to love myself.

I set boundaries that were more like walls because they weren't put there out of forgiveness and love of others, they were created out of my attempt at self-love manifesting as self-protection and fear. I was self-indulgent with my self-care. I believed that if I felt off, the right thing to do was just say no, just don't go, keeping in mind I need to come first. I have to fill my cup, or I can't fill others. The self-help, self-healing part of the modern world's culture tells me that I am doing it right. I am sitting in a bubble bath canceling on people I committed to in the name of self-love and filling my cup. I will help them tomorrow when my cup is full.

The question I had to ask myself was whether the journey to self-love had really brought me any lasting peace—not momentary peace, but lasting peace. Was I on an upward trajectory, one on which I could see where I was going and the positive impact it was having on my life and on the lives of those around me? Honestly, not at all. And for me, the journey ended up leaving me more self-focused than ever. I was focused on loving my body at every size. I was focused on trying to make sure my cup was full. My self-love practice is...fill in the blank. Me. Me. Me. In short, I was focused on making decisions based on what I believed would be best for me.

This led to an endless search for a self-love that I believed I felt occasionally, but it was mostly more like a never-ending race to a finish line that never arrived. Some days were better than others, but in the depths of my being, alone at night, I knew that something was off, but I wasn't sure what was missing.

I came to understand that my problem was that self-love was my goal when it is just the flip side of the self-consciousness coin. Self-love and being self-conscious are the two ends of the self-obsession pendulum, and there isn't real peace at either end. In the end, the answer was neither self-consciousness nor self-love, not self-doubt nor self-esteem, but *self-forgetting*. When I aimed toward self-love, I was still aiming at self, and I ended up at best subtly trying to overcompensate for the lack of peace I felt by faking it until I made it, and at worst, experiencing full-on panic and despair.

When I aimed toward self-forgetting, a whole new view began to open. Today, when it comes to my mind, I ask for help from God to direct my thinking back to the plans that He has in store for me. That might possibly mean time alone watching the latest thing on Netflix or a bubble bath, but I have found that is rarely what is asked of me. This does not mean I must give of myself to prove my love for others or that I am a self-sacrificial martyr. That route leads only to exhaustion, as my worth then depends on approval from the others for whom I am sacrificing. That is nowhere near true self-forgetting.

True self-forgetting happens in a place of willingness. I must have the willingness to stop and listen to the still small voice inside that lets me know whether to be alone or to reach out to help others. How I feel isn't in play at all, nor is my weight, my image, my clothes, my financial situation, my comfort, my approval from others, whether others love me, or whether others understand me. None of it comes to mind. There, I find true self-forgetting and true peace. So, I don't love myself, I also don't not love myself, I mostly just don't come to mind, and when I do, I pray. Let me tell you, it's a beautiful place to be.

Lesson 35

The True Nature of Negative Emotions

There was a time in my life when I looked back and I wished that things could have been different. I wished that my parents had not divorced. I wished that I had been born into a family with more money. I wished that I had been better at making friends. I wished that my friend had not been murdered. I wished that my high school boyfriend had not cheated on me. I wished I would have won that cross-country race in high school. I wished I had received an invitation to join from that one sorority in college. I wished that I had been admitted to that one college. I wished that a car accident had not killed those girls in college. I was sitting around wishing that I had been dealt a different hand in life. I thought that if I had, maybe things would be different, and maybe I would feel better.

But it was more than wishes about the past. I had wishes that were about the future as well. I wished that I would find the right husband. I wished for a big house. I wished for a higher paying job, or for a husband who made enough money that I did not have to work, or both. I wished for different friends and for more friends. I wished for more Instagram followers. I thought that if I had these things, maybe things would be different, maybe I would feel better.

All of this left me feeling overwhelmed, hopeless, and in despair. My negative emotions were at an all-time high. But the experience taught me a lot, both about negative emotions and about wishes. Without wishes, I wouldn't have negative emotions. Read that again. Without wishes, I would not have negative emotions.

Negative emotions always result from my wishes not being met. Whether I am experiencing sadness, anger, shame, remorse, regret, or any other negative emotion, it's always because of a wish. And some of the most overwhelming negative emotions are no different; they result from my continued frustration that my wishes are not being met. Hopelessness came from the feeling that my wishes consistently were not being met, and despair came from the feeling that they never would be met.

Why was I sad about the death or the break-up? My wish that they would be in my life forever, or at least for longer, did not come true. Why did I feel shame? My wish that this or that shameful thing was not true had not been granted. Why did I feel remorse or regret? Because of my wish that this or that terrible thing had not happened. So, if negative emotions were caused by these wishes, because of these demands that I unknowingly yet unfailingly placed on my life, what was I to do? Perhaps the obvious answer would be to reduce these wishes, these demands that I place on my life, because without them, I would have no negative emotions. But how am I to reduce these demands on and wishes for my life? The answer, in essence, is that I can't.

The only way to do it is to trust God.

I had to look back on my life and see that nothing in this world had ever truly filled me with joy the way I imagined it would, not the boy, the PhD, the job, the family relationships, the friendships, or the vacation. Put differently, nothing that I'd ever expected to be fulfilling had truly brought me unending happiness. If getting Prince Charming is the key to my happiness, what happens when Prince Charming disappoints me or dies? What happens when I am miserable in my mansion? You don't have to look far into either your own life or the lives of celebrities to see that there is nothing that makes one inherently and eternally happy. People who appear to have it all are often still filled with anxiety and may even resort to suicide.

Rather than looking to the world to fulfill my wishes, I now look to God to *reduce* them.

In other words, what has reduced my experience of negative emotions more than anything is to reduce my wishes and demands by turning my will and my life over to the care of God. It is only by daily obedience of God through acts of Faith that I find fulfillment. I ask God for help to trust His will for my life rather than my wishes for my life. And, the more fulfillment I find in God, the fewer demands I have for my life.

Some people will tell you that the key to experiencing fewer negative emotions is an attitude of gratitude, but I have found that gratitude band-aids and toxic positivity are nothing in comparison to the joy and peace that come from knowing that nothing I could ever wish for compares to God's plan for my life. I don't have to pretend that being grateful I have a roof over my head solves the current problems in my life. I can turn my negative emotions over to the care of God and then look back and see how each and every detail of my life has been used for good. I will never say that I needed the cards that I was dealt in order to be of use to God today, because God could have utilized any hand of cards. But I can see that He has indeed used each card for good.

So today, I know for sure that God can make use of any hand of cards for good if I let Him. When I don't allow for that, I end up drifting into a never-ending cloud of negative emotions, blaming the tribulations of my life for my negative feelings rather than recognizing them for what they are. They are simple indicators that I am living under the delusion that my wishes will make a better life for me than God's plan for my life. The truth is, most of my wishes are not even mine, they are just relics of familial and societal brainwashing. When I can let all of that go and trust God, no matter the tribulation, I get to live in peace, knowing that God will, in the fullness of time, use all things for good.

Lesson 36

God's Will Is Always Better than Mine

I recently went to the funeral of a woman I'd known; along with her husband, she had caused some pretty extreme disturbance in my life, as well as that of my boyfriend at the time (who is now my husband) and several of my family members. At the peak of the mayhem, everyone around me, including the police in my local area, thought my boyfriend and I should press charges and get a restraining order.

However, this whole situation unfolded right in the midst of my spiritual awakening and the time when I came to understand that the will of God is love. This is not to say that I don't believe in pressing charges when necessary, but in this case, I knew that love was the answer. I chose love. Rather than pressing charges, I prayed and prayed for the willingness to forgive them, as well as for my own wrong, which was my resentment toward them. It wasn't immediate, but it worked.

By 'it worked,' I don't mean they stopped harming us. They did cause one more major disturbance. But interestingly, although it was objectively just as problematic, it didn't have the same effect on me as on previous occasions, and my prayers worked much faster.

Their behavior was the catalyst for one of my first lessons in following God's will. By choosing God's will, which was to forgive and love rather than to separate and hate, I found peace. That's what I mean when I say it worked. I do believe that even if I had felt called to press charges, the only way to find peace still would have been to forgive and to seek healing for any resentment that I had, even in the midst of necessary legal action.

Moreover, I have found that when I have run into this man and his wife over the last few years, I am always able to calmly say hello without anxiety or panic. They never made amends, and although she obviously cannot make amends after her recent death, he still probably never will. However, my forgiveness doesn't require them to be sorry, it just requires that I choose to live in love rather than in justified anger. I believe this is the will of God, and at her funeral, I prayed that her soul rests in peace. In fact, as odd as it sounds, what she and her husband did a few years ago didn't even come to mind until I began to write this essay.

Over the past couple of years, I have found that when I become aware of and follow the will of God, it always eventually brings serenity, and when I don't, it always eventually brings suffering of some kind. In some situations, God's will might be obvious, for example, not cheating or lying when tempted. Honesty is love, cheating and lying are not. At other times, God's will, although clear, isn't so obvious in terms of its morality in application.

Here's an example. My husband (then my fiancé) and I were on a Caribbean cruise over the holidays in 2022. On the first night, Christmas Eve, we ate in the Tuscan restaurant on the ship, where we had a gracious server named Alexio. The following night, the ship offered a midnight Christmas service, which we attended. Later that week, we somehow decided that out of all the restaurants on the ship, we wanted to go back to the Tuscan restaurant. We were once again seated in Alexio's section, and he mentioned he had seen us in the service. We connected immediately. We talked about faith and about his wife, Liza, and his three daughters back in India. He found out that we were engaged and told us to come back the final night of the cruise for a special engagement dessert.

The last day on the ship, they had a raffle for a pair of diamond earrings. At the last minute, I decided to enter the raffle, and to my surprise, I won. I was so excited to wear the earrings to dinner that last night on the ship. As I was getting ready to put them on, the voice of God came in as loud and clear as though it was in my head, but emanating from my heart. The earrings were for Alexio's wife, Liza, not for me. I prayed to be sure, but I already knew.

I could feel the peace in my heart at the thought of giving them to Liza, and I could feel the suffering that would result from choosing to ignore that still small voice from inside. My thinking mind even tried to stop me, "But what about my sister, or my mother? Shouldn't I give the earrings to them if I am going to give them away?" But God's will is not rational, God's will is love, and deep down I knew what His will was for me that night.

I gave the earrings to Alexio at dinner, and he burst into tears. I know it was God's will. I know that was an act of love. I know that God is love. I may never know why that was God's will, but I know the peace that came from following it.

My only resolution this year is to stay in God's will, which means to stay in love, not with myself, but with God and with others, because as Saint Francis of Assisi said in his famous prayer, "It is by self-forgetting that one finds. It is by forgiving that one is forgiven. It is by dying that one awakens to Eternal Life." This means not dying a physical death but dying to my own self-will and waking up to the eternal peace of God's will. Living in love means putting God's will first. By doing so, I have been given a second chance at life. This second round is full of faith, love, and forgiveness, and it is available to anyone who seeks it. Today is a great day to start.

Lesson 37

The Real Secret to Happiness

Let me start with a question someone once asked me.

"Do you believe that you would be happier if something about the world or about someone else in the world was different?"

If you answered yes, you are living in a delusion, and you are probably unhappy, just as I was.

For most of my life, I believed that if "they" would change, things would be different. If the world was different, if I was dealt different cards, then I would be happy. As I was drifting into a nap earlier today, I was thinking about some of the beautiful things that are true about my life today that happened because I let God take the lead in my life.

I live in a beautiful townhouse with my husband, who loves me dearly. I get to ride a motorcycle all summer here in Minnesota in beautiful weather. My social life is full of plans with people who really mean something to me. I have a flexible schedule and get to travel quite a bit. I see my family several times a year even though they live halfway across the country. I have a close group of girlfriends. I am learning how to wakesurf this summer. Is this why I am happy? Absolutely not.

Do you want to know why? What if I had drifted into my nap thinking about my life in a different way? I live in a rented townhouse when other people my age live in homes they bought. My husband has an annoying sense of humor at times and way too many motorcycles. Other men are often better at humor and spend money on more important things. My schedule has been too busy to be able to motorcycle much this summer. I got laid off from my job last year. Now, I don't know what I am going to do next or how I am going to replace that income. Everyone just drinks all the time on summer weekends in Minnesota. My Instagram account isn't growing very fast. I met most of my close girlfriends in recovery, so they could relapse at any time. I try to wakesurf with my friends, but I am not as good at it as all of them are.

I did not change any facts about my life to write that last paragraph above. What I changed was my reaction to the world and to the people around me. I became a victim of others. Wishing that the world was different or that people were different will always be the main source of human unhappiness. Believing that change that takes place outside of me will cause me to be happy is the core delusion of all humanity.

The following is a little example loosely borrowed from Anthony DeMello, a Jesuit speaker. When it comes to another person, wishing that *they* were different is like going to the doctor and saying, "I have an infection," and the doctor telling you, "Okay, let me prescribe some medication for your neighbor to see if it helps your infection go away." We would think that was absurd because the infection is not in my neighbor, the infection and the pain are in me.

However, people do this all the time as it relates to their happiness, and they don't see it as absurd. When I say, "I wish that my husband would see that his humor sometimes offends people," that is me saying that I wish the doctor would prescribe something for him, then I can be happy. Society tells us that this is normal, but reacting this way is absurd. The pain I am suffering from is my judgment of him, along with my fear of losing approval from others. His humor is not the problem, my judgment and fear are the problem for me. When I can see this clearly and know that it is my fault, not his fault—that it is fully my fault—I can bring my wrongs to God and watch the pain fall away in the face of my newfound humility.

My friends and I have a funny little saying that we tell each other to remind ourselves of this. When someone does something mean, rude, harmful, or the like, most people would say, "They hurt my feelings." We say, "I hurt my own feelings today." It applies to everything. The last time I had a boyfriend cheat on me, he did not hurt my feelings. Luckily, he does not have the power to do that. The truth is, I hurt my own feelings. He did something I perceived as awful, so I gave myself a bad feeling.

So, what do I do about this? I start by recognizing that the bad feeling is always in me, not in another person and not in the world. When I can do that, I begin to see clearly that my feeling of unhappiness is not a result of the outside world being different than the way I want it to be. Instead, the outside world appearing to not be the way I want it to be is a result of me feeling unhappiness. Therefore, happiness results from dropping the delusion that happiness comes from the outside in and realizing that it comes from the inside out.

Lesson 38

I Don't Want to Be Confident

I used to wish I had more self-confidence. I would watch people effortlessly walk into parties and social settings and talk to anyone. I watched people pitch business ideas with ease. I saw people ace every question in interviews. I watched people who always looked stylish and put together even when they were seemingly not trying. I wished to be as self-confident as they were or at least appeared to be.

Then I realized two things, the first of which is less important, but I will share it first simply to get it out of the way. Watching someone else's behavior does not tell me much about what is going on inside of them. This is ever more true as psychiatric medication and self-medication with drugs and alcohol have become normalized. I do not know if someone else is confident or nervous, nor whether their current state is artificially induced or organic. But that is the less important insight.

The more important insight is that I was wishing for the wrong states of mind all along. I wished to be self-confident, to be confident in myself. To me, that meant, for example, that I was would be confident that I was making a good impression, confident that I sounded intelligent, confident that I looked amazing, or confident because I was well-prepared or well-educated. I wanted this because I had spent so much time in a state in which I was lacking confidence, also known as self-consciousness. I was nervous that I was not making a good impression or not sounding intelligent, worried that I did not look amazing or even how I hoped I would look, or anxious that I was underprepared or not educated enough.

True freedom does not come from either of these states of mind. Self-confidence is just the opposite end of self-consciousness; they both indicate self-absorption. Self-consciousness is judging myself with disapproval or believing that others are disapproving of me. Self-confidence is judging myself in an approving way or living in the delusion that I am getting approval from others. These states were setting me up for some kind of pain because I could not just "be," I was always in a state of performance. Self-forgetting is freedom from it all.

Currently, I neither want to be confident that I am making a good impression nor fearful of making a bad one; I would rather have no awareness of needing to make an impression at all. I do not want to be confident that I sound intelligent or fearful that I don't, for true peace is the state of not being aware of needing to sound any particular way. I do not want to be confident that I look amazing or fearful that I don't, I just don't want to be aware of how I think I look, nor how anyone else thinks I look.

Here's an example that might help emphasize this. Imagine that it's my birthday, and that I feel self-conscious about how I look. So, I say to my partner, "I am really feeling self-conscious about how I look." Imagine he says, "Honey, you have never looked better. I cannot even believe you would say that!" Now, we have relieved the pain of my self-consciousness and maybe even propelled me into self-confidence.

Now imagine that I walk away, and he then turns to our friend and says, "I couldn't bring myself to tell her she looks awful." Since I never find out what he really thinks nor what he said, I live out the rest of the day confident as can be and in complete delusion. At the end of the day, if I find out he was lying, it all flips on its head. Instead, what if I had just not worried about it at all? What if I had not judged myself as looking either good or bad, nor worried about what anyone else thought?

That's peace, and it's far better than confidence. Confidence depends on my belief that I am performing well; peace is not thinking about the performance at all, it's just being.

Where self-confidence shows up forcefully and says, "I am important," self-forgetting shows up and just says, "I am here." Where self-confidence is me trying to force myself to be happy with the shape and size of my body, self-forgetting is me not thinking about my body at all. Self-confidence is believing I know just as much as the next person; self-forgetting is not assessing how much either of us know. Self-confidence is planning for the perfect execution; self-forgetting is prayerfully doing the next right thing.

The bridge from the island of self-confidence and self-consciousness to the shore of self-forgetting is made of self-examination and prayer. Today, I live more of my life than not in a state of self-forgetting. Getting to the shore of self-forgetting was not an overnight matter. When I become aware of my own self-consciousness or self-confidence, I pray for God's will instead, for freedom from the bondage of self. I always used to wonder why people asked God to take the good and the bad, but now I see that if I want to live in peace, I want God to take it all. The excitement of self-confidence is not worth the pain of self-consciousness, and it isn't nearly as freeing as the joy of self-forgetting.

Lesson 39

Stop Trying to Control Outcomes

Giving up control to God can seem daunting at first, but there's good news. Living in faith is not about me giving up control to God because I never had any to begin with. Instead, it's about giving up the illusion of control. Unfortunately, I was slow to learn this lesson.

For example, I spent much of my life trying to control my health while in a constant state of chronic illness. I had terrible IBS. I had gastric dumping that a doctor once described as the worst he had seen outside of botched gastric bypass patients. I thought I had gluten and dairy intolerance as well as a number of other less common food intolerances because I was having seemingly random debilitating stomach aches. I was chronically tired. I sometimes broke out in full body hives. I was diagnosed with alopecia areata when I developed six unexplained bald spots. I had chronic UTIs and a recurring stye in one of my eyes. There were probably other health conditions, but that's all I can remember now.

I desperately wanted all of this to change. I tried different diets, medications, doctors, alternative medicines, and more, all without prayer or direction from God. I was always going to control myself better the next day—the "Magic Pillow Cure." You may be familiar with it. The Magic Pillow Cure is the belief that I will be able to change tomorrow what I could not change today. In other words, it is the belief that there is something magical about placing my head on my pillow and getting a little sleep. It sounds silly written out this way, but anyone who has ever said, "My diet starts tomorrow!" has engaged in this exact type of thinking—that I can control tomorrow what I have never been able to control before, that I'll do this or that tomorrow and then things will be different.

Today, I know that I cannot control outcomes. The only thing I have control over is whether I turn the next behavior over to God and am willing to follow God's will in doing the next right thing. If the actions I am taking today are only in service of a certain desired outcome and not in service of God's will for me today, I am bound to be disappointed when something inevitably does not go my way.

I can look back and see that I could not ever force an outcome in the long term. In the short term, it sometimes appeared that I had control. But in the long run, I have never found this to be true. Have you ever lost weight and gained it back? Have you ever heard of a person who exercises regularly but still suffers from a random heart attack or cancer? I can try to control outcomes, but I never really have control.

Furthermore, I am faced with the fact that anything I want to control has taken the place of God for me. If I need better health, health is god. If I need more money, money is god. If I need more ambition, ambition is god. God does not want me to improve myself in the way I see fit, He wants me to surrender to life as He sees fit. What's surprising is that's where happiness is revealed.

The outcomes that I was so desperately trying to force never actually made me happy. Was there excitement? Sure. Was there sensate pleasure? Sure. But was there the happiness of true fulfillment in life? There was not. At its core, my need for control was an addiction to hearing "attagirl" for attaining certain outcomes. But as long as I was trying to attain happiness through either an internal or external "attagirl" instead of by surrendering my will to God, I was never going to truly be fulfilled, even if that "attagirl" was an internal congratulations to myself that I ate healthy or stayed sober. If I did it and left God out, I was inevitably setting myself up for disappointment rather than fulfillment.

In the end, the illusion of control cannot live in a heart that is fully surrendered to God. A heart full of God is incompatible with the need to control outcomes. And it's much simpler than it seems, because my job is not to decide what outcomes God wants and to strive for them. My job is just to do what God asks and then let the outcomes unfold as they do.

For the record, one day at a time, my hair grew back, I am no longer intolerant of any foods, I don't break out in hives, I am not chronically exhausted, I am not on any medications, and I can't remember the last time I had a debilitating stomachache. All of that happened by following God's will where it took me, not by trying to change myself.

Lesson 40

Expressing My Emotions to Others Isn't Healing

In December of 2021, I was on a motorcycle trip with my then boyfriend, now husband, Kevin, and two of our friends, Elliot and Peter. We were in Mexico headed back toward the United States, only a few hours from the border. Elliot was leading us, followed by Peter, me, and Kevin, in that order. We were on a long straight road, common in rural Mexico. All of a sudden, there was a sharp left turn in the road. Elliot went through the turn, and although he had to hit the brakes, he did make the turn. Peter was behind him. Unfortunately, Peter hit gravel and did not make the turn. I was third, which meant that I had a front row seat to the wreckage as Peter's bike and body flew up into the air, and for a split second, I was sure that I was going to face the same fate.

However, I hit the brakes, made the turn, and rolled to a stop about a hundred meters down the road. I parked, got off my bike, and saw pieces of Peter's motorcycle strewn about the road. His body was lying in a rocky roadside ditch. I could hear him groaning, so I knew he wasn't dead. He was transported to the nearest hospital, about an hour away, by a medic unit for a construction crew that happened to be doing work down the road. We had called an ambulance that was on its way, but it was going to be an hour before it arrived, and we decided that time might be important. Elliot followed the medics while Kevin and I found a way to load most of Peter's luggage onto our motorcycles, although we were forced to leave the less important items behind.

As it became time to get back on the motorcycles and head toward the hospital, the fight-or-flight condition in which I had been functioning began to wear off and fear came up, and I reacted to it by expressing it. I stood beside my motorcycle and told Kevin I was full of fear and that I wasn't getting on my bike. I said that I didn't want to keep going and that I actually never wanted to ride again, all of which was true at that moment.

He just looked at me. I had expressed how I felt at that moment, but it was neither particularly useful nor healing. Non-reactive fellow that he is, he said, "Okay, no problem. How are you going to get home, and what's your plan for getting your motorcycle and luggage home, should you want to keep those?" I had no plan, and, of course, I did want my luggage. I took a deep breath and suppressed my feelings. My feelings may have been valid, but they were not useful, and I had always been good at stuffing them. So, that's what I did as we made the one-hour ride to the hospital.

When we arrived, we found that Peter was not in good condition. He was not going to die, but he had a lot of broken bones—eleven to be exact, from his shoulders down. The first few hours at the hospital were confusing. We had to figure out Peter's insurance. There were language barriers. There was a lack of trust on both ends. The hospital wanted photos of the accident to prove we had not just beat him up. They wanted to know why the medics had brought him rather than the ambulance. It was mayhem. I was getting angrier and angrier as they delayed his treatment until these issues were resolved. And it was getting later and darker outside. I stayed calm by suppressing everything I felt.

That night as I was lying in bed, everything finally hit me. I was angry that Peter had not made the turn. I was angry that Elliot hadn't seen it coming. I feared motorcycling after seeing Peter's accident. I was scared Peter wouldn't get appropriate treatment at the hospital. I was angry at the Mexican medical system for putting finances before treatment. I had suppressed those emotions much of the day. I had expressed my fear before I got on the bike, and I had expressed some anger to the staff at the hospital as well, but I had not done the one thing that would actually help: confession.

The "gift" of suppressing emotions is that they come back. The "gift" of simply expressing them is that it only provides temporary relief, at most. When I use either expression or suppression, the feelings gnaw and wait to be truly healed. Telling someone I am angry is not the solution for being angry. Telling someone I am fearful is not the solution to being fearful. Sometimes it actually becomes worse if they tell me that my feelings are valid, and I begin to grow pride around their validity.

The solution is confessing them first to myself, then to God, and when they are really gnawing, to another human being—not that I am angry or fearful, but that I am wrong for being angry and fearful. For me, lasting peace has never come from expressing my emotions to another person, it has come by confessing them. "I am angry" or "I am so scared" are expressions. "God forgive me for my anger" or "God, help, I know I am wrong for this anger" or "God, take away my fear and show me what you would have me be" are all confessions.

True healing does not happen when I express emotions such as anger or fear, nor when I suppress them. It comes by confessing that I know that anger is not the path, and that fear will not serve me because these emotions are not in alignment with Divine Love. It doesn't mean that I am bad for having them, it just means they are indicators that I need God's help, not that I need to tell someone how I feel. That night in

Mexico, I confessed my anger and my fear to God, and when I woke up
the next morning, the situation looked a lot different to me. I wasn't
afraid of what would happen to Peter. I wasn't angry at the hospital nor
the staff. And I was not afraid to hop right back on my motorcycle that
day, nor on any day since.

Lesson 41

The Truth about Low Self-Esteem

For as long as I can remember, I have been introspective. I have spent a lot of time thinking and wondering about myself and other people. I have not only wondered about life, but also wondered why I felt different. It seemed easier for other kids to get along with one another and play. It wasn't so easy for me. In preschool, I was more comfortable spending time with my teachers than with the other kids. In kindergarten, my favorite play station was the writing station where I could journal. I liked organized sports because there were specific rules of engagement. It did not require me to just figure out how to interact with other people.

For most of elementary school, I struggled to make friends. I had one close friend for most of that time. I was sure that she was my friend. As for everyone else, I couldn't figure them out. Here is the weird part though. Looking back, there are a lot of people from that time who probably would have called me their friend, but my self-consciousness just got in the way of me realizing it.

In middle school, high school, and college, I always had a friend group, but I always felt less-than compared to others. I felt as though fitting in was more difficult for me than for other people. I was constantly worried about saying or doing the wrong thing and suddenly being left out. I would catastrophize even small negative situations, worrying that they were the end of my social life. I always worried that at best, people were noticing that I wasn't fitting in, or at worst, not noticing me at all.

I tried to make up for my insecurity by achieving. I tried to get straight A's and mostly did so. I tried to excel in sports. Although it was a rare occurrence, when I did not make the team, the starting line-up, or the top spot on the honor roll, I was devastated. I couldn't have told you why at the time, but looking back, it was because my self-worth was wrapped up in the outside world. I was living in fear, fear that I was not enough and never would be.

At the time, I thought I just had low self-esteem, social anxiety, generalized anxiety, plus maybe a little depression, or maybe I was just socially awkward and different. But what was my real problem? I was constantly ruminating on myself.

I once read somewhere that high and low self-esteem come from the same place; that is, they are both prideful. It's funny, because if someone had told me that my low self-esteem and my insecurity were pride, I would have told them there was no way that was so. But that day, when I read it, it hit me that it was. Pride is rumination on the self, self-absorption. Whether that self-absorption results in a delusionally high or a delusionally low opinion of oneself is just a matter of the content, but the spiritual nature of the problem was the same for me: I was self-absorbed.

I was ruminating on myself and deciding that everything I observed was a flaw. The result was low self-esteem and insecurity. I worried what everyone was thinking about me. The key words there are "about me." If I had just been genuinely interested in what others were thinking, it wouldn't have resulted in the same hit to my self-esteem because it wouldn't have been about me.

My problem was self-saturation, and my self-saturation was the result of separation from God caused by my pride. As odd as it is to say, recovery from this state of low self-esteem was not a result of reminding myself that I am enough. That would just swing the pendulum to the other pole of the pride duality yet leave me self-saturated. Recovery came by confessing my pride repeatedly and letting God change my heart, which, in turn, changed my mind to the point that I don't worry anymore whether I am enough or not enough, I just exist.

So now, whenever I find myself in a state of self-consciousness or low self-esteem, I ask God to forgive me for my pride and self-saturation to relieve me of my selfishness—and slowly but surely, it continues to work. I never would have believed you if you had told me that low-self-esteem was selfishness and pride, but my experience is that when I confess it as such, the result is relief from low self-esteem. I didn't end up with high self-esteem, what I got was relief from constant internal assessment of my self-esteem and a closer connection with God.

Lesson 42

Setting Boundaries Is Not a Panacea

I used to say, "I feel so selfish for setting these boundaries." People deep in the self-help world would assure me that I was on the right track, and so I continued. These same people say, "The boundary is just for me." Meanwhile, the boundary may be something like, "If you are going to drink, then I am going to remove myself from the situation," or "If you call me a mean name, I will not participate in arguments with you." This is not just for a given situation, a boundary is setting the expectation for the rules of engagement. And yes, when I do this, I am not telling the other person what to do per se, but I almost always create a situation in which I am in essence giving an ultimatum, and then calling it my own boundary. I am saying that because I set this rule, if you behave in a way that breaks it and that messes with my peace of mind, you do not get to be in a relationship with me, and I have no fault. The fault is yours because I set the rules and you broke them.

I know some people may be challenged by this, but boundaries are always inherently selfish, and no, not in a good way. Why? Because they are set in fear. Now, if you have a new type of boundary that is something different than the boundaries I speak of here, you'll have to ask yourself if this is true for you. But I do hope you'll keep an open mind to the fact that no matter how loving you hope it is, it might, in fact, be selfishly set in fear.

We set boundaries because we are fearful of others. We are not able to control things. We become discontent. We get irritable. Perhaps we are trying to avoid becoming passive-aggressive, so we set a boundary.

Boundaries put the focus on external protection as a means of keeping a dubious sort of peace of mind. We are like little dictators, saying that if only everyone would behave just as I want, then everything would be great and no one, including me, would ever be upset.

That sounds great, right? Wrong. My husband always likes to say, "You know why they push your buttons?" He will wait while the person ponders and then say, "It's because you have buttons installed." It's not because I was in a toxic relationship, although sometimes I was. It's not because they were toxic, although maybe they were. It is not because they were committing wrongdoing against me, although maybe they were. All of those may be true, but 100 percent of the time, when I am triggered, it is because I have a trigger button installed within myself that got pushed.

The irony of boundaries is they are a form of protection from people pushing my buttons, when the problem is not their pushing but that I have a button. Someone pushing the button might be the best gift I have ever been given because I get a chance to recognize that I have a button and can take the time to examine the nature of that button so that I can remove it. Getting a button pushed is a chance to see where I can still grow spiritually. It is a chance to love in a new way. It is a chance to see how controlling I really am. It is a chance to see how many expectations I have of other people. It is a chance to notice how I still judge others.

Boundaries may create temporary peace of mind, but peace of soul does not come from external consistency created by keeping people away from us or making them act in certain ways around us. Peace of soul comes from asking God to remove the buttons so that I am unaffected by the behavior of those around me. Loving others does not require boundaries. It requires communication, yes. But it never requires hard and fast rules of engagement. In response to this idea, you might say, "I am open to changing my boundary." Sure, I used to say that, too. However, that is not the point.

The point is that God's will for me is always to examine my own judgments of others and clear the channel so I can see how I can serve others. God's will for me is never to protect myself from disturbance or judge another person's behavior as wrong. That means that my first line of action in difficult times is always to hit my knees and pray. First, I ask God's forgiveness for my resentment, fear, and judgment. When I feel disturbed, I am usually guilty of all three. I then ask for insight into how I might have caused the situation to develop. It is *never* just the other person who is at fault. It is never just because they are controlling, irresponsible, or a narcissist, as much as I want to believe it is when I am living in fear instead of faith.

So, I pray until I see my faults. I even ask for insight into my history to see if unforgiven past resentments might be the cause of my present disturbance. With deep resentment, I almost always need to look back to childhood to ask God to remove all past resentment there. I am only ready to communicate with the other person when I see all my faults and no longer hold resentment, past or present—in other words, not until I have dismantled the trigger button.

Only once I have done all this am I ready to communicate, and here is the irony. When I do this, I realize that I do not need to make rules of engagement—that I was just living in resentment, which produced the fear and need for control I was experiencing. It does not mean that person must be first on my list of people to spend time with, but I do not have to make up hard and fast rules. I can live in the moment. Not only that, but I also realize the disturbance was actually a beautiful opportunity to grow spiritually. I was given the chance to remove a trigger button, or at least take part of it out. I now realize that boundaries were truly my foe because they only led to temporary peace of mind. And I know that triggers are my friend, because they are the path to button removal and consistent, trigger-button-free peace of soul.

Lesson 43

You Cannot Transmit an Awakening You Haven't Had

One of the main realizations I have had in adulthood is that therapists are broken people, just like the rest of us. So why do we go to them for help? We go because they offer tools to lessen the pain, tools for coping, and tools for tapping into our forgotten memories and the unconscious. Unlike spiritual guidance, therapists are not transmitting grace or peace, they are offering suggestions and helping us see the patterns. They usually aren't trying to allow God to speak through them.

As a result, they can help, at least to a certain degree, regardless of what is going on inside of them. They can offer suggestions to me to improve my marriage even if theirs is falling apart. They can offer tools to help me navigate a family holiday even if they resent their own family. When a spiritual mentor is acting as a junior therapist instead of as a spiritual mentor, they, too, can help me to a certain degree, regardless of what is going on inside of them. But in my experience, they couldn't get me where I really needed to go because they were trying to teach me psychological tools rather than lead me to a spiritual awakening.

Physicians function in the same way. You can have a very sick yet effective doctor. Doctors can have a wealth of knowledge, for example, about diabetes or heart disease that is useful to you regardless of whether they take care of their own health. A doctor with bad knees can still perform an effective knee surgery.

When it comes to spirituality, this is not how it works. In spirituality, I cannot transmit something I don't have. I cannot show up full of my own anger, fear, jealousy, judgment, and the like, expecting to help relieve you of yours. I have tried—not on purpose, of course—but looking back, there have been moments when I was not doing the work because of my excuses, and it showed up in my ability to help others. Why? Because in spirituality, you cannot transmit faith that you aren't living in yourself.

If I haven't forgiven my parents for their divorce, I cannot help you forgive yours. If I think it's fine to hate the people who have harmed me, I can't help you love others unconditionally. If I am jealous of people living life differently than me, I can't help you see the beauty in your day-to-day life. If I believe this or that should have happened, I can't help you accept life on life's terms. If I harm others and say, "It's because I am only human" rather than seeing how I am wrong, I can expect to have a mentee full of excuses rather than faith. Every single time, my excuses as a mentor will get in the way of your spiritual awakening as a mentee.

In fact, in my experience, a spiritual mentor can only help you up to the point of their own excuses. They may not even realize they have these excuses, but everyone has a place where they just haven't gone yet, and if I haven't gone to that place, God can't help me lead you there. If I choose a spiritual mentor full of excuses, I will continue to suffer, whether I am aware of it or not. Oddly, sometimes suffering felt like comfort because I was so used to suffering. One of my early mentors told me that some people do unforgivable things. If what they did was bad enough, if it harmed me enough, then I did not have to forgive. I stayed comfortably in the belief that I could hold resentment, and I also stayed sick, mentally, physically, and spiritually.

She was not a bad person. She had the ability to choose to not forgive and stay sober. She was comfortable where she was; she just didn't want to binge drink. As such, that was the threshold for her excuses. "I am sober, and I didn't have to forgive, so you can stay sober and not forgive." However, I wanted more in my life than another day free from binge drinking, so I needed a different mentor. She could transmit that level of healing to me but nothing more, so I needed a new mentor if I wanted to be at peace with everyone and everything. Her excuses would have kept me from continuing my own awakening.

Today, I have mentors who push me to unconditional love, unconditional forgiveness, and unconditional faith. They challenge me to dig deeper and question every nook and cranny of my resentments, fears, and habits. Most recently, I have been challenging my belief that anything in life should be fair. To believe that life should be fair was an excuse for resentment and fear that was keeping me sick.

Today, I get to be that mentor for others. The gift of being a mentor keeps me forever on the path of identifying and challenging my own excuses and giving them up to God, so that my excuses never stand in the way of someone else's awakening. It's a daily practice, but it is so worth it to move closer and closer to complete union with God, because there is no better feeling than watching another person wake up and heal.

PART IV

Radical Forgiveness

Lesson 44

I Had Forgiveness All Wrong

I used to struggle with being angry and fearful about the prospect of unconditional forgiveness. I was angry when people suggested that unconditional forgiveness is an option for everyone, regardless of what others have done to them. *Clearly, they didn't know my history.* Moreover, I was fearful that if I forgave people who had abused me or harmed me, I would be setting myself up to be hurt again. As it turns out, this is a common but profound misunderstanding of forgiveness.

Let me try to explain this misunderstanding of forgiveness with a metaphor. Imagine that you are holding a fishing rod, and at the end of your fishing line there is a fish on a hook. The fish is the person I am choosing not to forgive, and the hook and line are the unforgiveness and resentment. When I choose not to forgive someone, I am choosing to leave the hook in the fish and hold tight to the line. No matter where it goes, I am attached to it. Some days the line might be loose, and I may barely notice the tug at all, but on other days, it is tight, and I am constantly "triggered" or in a state of anxiety.

When I used to think of forgiveness, I thought that what was being asked of me was to reel in the fish and give it a hug. That is not forgiveness. Forgiveness is letting go of the fishing line.

Forgiveness does not even require that I contact the other person. I don't have to let them know that I have forgiven them. In fact, the desire to let the other person know I forgave them can sometimes come from my own pride. Instead, forgiveness is looking to God and saying something like, "I am ready. I know they were suffering. Please help me forgive them." The words don't matter; prayer comes from the heart, not the mind. "Forgive them, they know not what they do," is just the essence. When I do this, I am not hugging the fish, I am letting go of the line. The fish can't tug on me at random. The grasp I let it have on me is over.

For me, what has always followed a prayer like this from the heart is a total transformation of my understanding of the other person. In some cases, that means that once I let go of the line, I can enjoy their company or have them in my life in some capacity. In other cases, there has been no further contact between me and the other person. But regardless of the outcome on the person-to-person level, true forgiveness is the release of the hook on the spiritual level.

Here's a pretty simple example. Last summer, my then fiancé, now husband, and I returned from a trip to find that someone had smashed the rear driver side window of our truck. One of the first things that I did after seeing the shattered window was sit down in the passenger seat and pray a prayer like the one above.

Complete forgiveness doesn't mean that I want the vandal to be my friend, but it does mean that I'm now living life without a hook of resentment and unforgiveness set in the vandal. It means that seeing a smashed car window will not automatically trigger this memory, and it means that if the memory does ever return, it will not come with negative emotion attached to it.

When I have forgiven, the memory only returns if I can use the story to be helpful to another person. If the memory is triggered and it comes with negative emotions, I have not yet forgiven, and I keep praying until I am ready to release the hook. God doesn't require multiple prayers from me on His end, but oftentimes, full release requires multiple prayers on my end before I am ready to let go of the hook.

Now for a more seemingly complicated example: forgiving my ex. The relationship in question included several physical arguments as well as a lot of other abusive behaviors. When I was ready, I got on my knees and asked God for help forgiving him and releasing my resentment toward him. After many prayers, when I finally turned all that over to God, I felt peace. However, I didn't feel the need to call him and tell him that I had let go of the hook, nor did I feel compelled to contact him at all, for that matter. The goal of forgiveness was not to get back together with him, the goal was to get free of the anger and unforgiveness that I was holding on to so that I could clearly see whether he belonged in my life or not.

When I am so clouded by anger that I can't even see the other person's humanity, when I can't remember that when I'm looking into their eyes, I am looking into the eyes of someone who, deep down, doesn't want to be in pain or harm others, I am in no position to make a decision about whether they should or should not be in my life. Only forgiveness allows me the clarity to make that decision.

I know that thinking about forgiveness can bring up anger and fear. To be honest, in some cases, I wasn't sure who I would be without resentment, without the chip on my shoulder, without being the victim. I would shout, "Those people knew what they were doing! Those people meant to harm me! Those people don't deserve my forgiveness." But deep down, I just wasn't sure who I would be after forgiveness. It turns out I am a much happier and more pleasant person to be around. Hooks of unforgiveness made me emotionally unpredictable and left me constantly seeking validation for my pain. Prayerful forgiveness has allowed me to see both myself and others through a clear and loving lens, no matter what they have done.

Lesson 45

Anyone Can Be Forgiven

When my husband, Kevin, got his last DUI before getting sober in the year 2000, he was required to attend a Mothers Against Drunk Driving (MADD) panel event as part of his sentencing. On MADD's website, it explains that at these panels, those affected by drunk driving talk "... about the crime's impact upon themselves, their families, friends, and the community as a whole. During the panel, speakers describe the crash in which they or their loved ones were involved, and how life has changed since the crash... Victim Impact Panels are designed to provide offenders with the understanding that drunk driving is a choice that impacts the lives of innocent people." Most of these panels involve individuals actively expressing anger and grief. Kevin, aware of his guilt and having accepted the consequences, braced himself for a display of resentment and gore.

The event began, and three individuals walked onto the stage, seemingly a mother, father, and son. The parents began describing a crash that had taken place a few years prior in which a drunk driver's behavior had resulted in the death of their sixteen-year-old daughter. They described the police coming to the door. When the father answered the door, he already knew something had happened because their daughter was generally responsible and home on time. He called to his wife, who came running down the stairs. The police described the situation to both of them. Another teenager had been driving drunk, and he had crashed into their daughter's motor vehicle. Their daughter was dead, but the drunk teenager, who had survived the crash with little injury, was in custody. The officer promised the bail would be set high. "How high?" the mom asked. "Very high, ma'am," the officer responded. "How high?" she repeated. He told her.

Unbeknownst to everyone else, she had already prayed, and God had already placed an unfathomable amount of forgiveness in her heart. She asked for a lower bail, which was of course granted. She used her own savings to bail the young man out of prison on the condition that he would come to live with them in their daughter's bedroom and would begin attending recovery meetings.

On stage, their "son" had remained quiet throughout the story. At this point, he stepped forward and revealed that the mother's profound forgiveness had changed his life. This was not the girl's brother but the teen who had killed her. Her mother had offered him forgiveness, and he now had several years of sobriety. The father described his anger toward his wife at first. He wanted to murder the boy, perhaps understandably, and yet the boy was living in his daughter's room at his wife's request. The boy had even stood with the mother at the wake and walked with her down the aisle at the daughter's funeral.

Eventually, by watching his wife's profound acts of faith, the father's heart softened. They'd lost a daughter, but they had a son.

Instead of moving into despair at the greatest pain they had ever experienced, they chose forgiveness and love, and it profoundly changed not only their own lives and the life of the boy, but now the lives of thousands of individuals across the country who heard their story, both firsthand at MADD panels and secondhand from those who attended those panels, myself included. Kevin said there was not a dry eye in the auditorium. Even the most hardened human hearts are moved at true forgiveness.

I will never know why Kevin got to experience that panel instead of having a more common, harsher MADD panel experience, but him telling me that story changed my life. I heard it in the midst of coming to understand that in order to recover, to experience true freedom from all my various addictions and mental illnesses, I had to be free from anger, and that meant unconditional forgiveness. There were instances of harm that others had caused me that I believed were unforgivable. Then I heard that story, and my heart softened. If she can do that, with God's help, so can I.

Forgiveness is a choice, and forgiveness is work. I have never done it successfully without prayer and God's help. But here is the biggest gift of forgiveness: I no longer live with the memories of harm done to me by others. In the past, I was someone who used to experience flashbacks at random; now, I am someone who basically forgets.

Forgive and forget or remember and hate. Forgiveness is not a matter of determining that what they did wasn't wrong, it's a matter of letting go of the memory and the pain. Today, those who have harmed me in the past do not come to mind except in one circumstance, when I sit down with another recovering person to help show them that forgiving and forgetting is possible. I have talked to others in recovery who have the same experience with forgiveness and memory. I never knew that it was truly possible to forgive and forget, but it is. The memory is gone, except when it comes back so that I can say, "That happened to me, too, and I promise you, with enough prayer, forgiveness is possible."

If the memory isn't gone, I don't fool myself into thinking that I have forgiven, because although I may want to forgive with my mind, it means I haven't forgiven from the heart, and it is an immediate sign for me to go back to prayer and dig deeper into forgiveness. It means some little part of me is still hanging onto unforgiveness. When I truly let go, the memory is gone, except when God brings it back to me so that I can carry the message to others that total forgiveness and total healing are possible.

Lesson 46

Saying "They Did the Best They Could" Is Still a Judgment

"I used to have so much unresolved confusion and anger about certain negative experiences from my childhood, like my parent's divorce, but eventually, I realized that my parents did the best they could." I used to say things like this, and I thought I was doing pretty well, perhaps even more awakened than the average Jane.

However, "They did the best they could" came out of my mouth one day in the presence of someone who had truly awakened. He looked me straight in the eyes and said, "Saying 'They did the best they could' is still a judgment. Just wake up and let go of it."

That one hit me hard. I was not ready to accept that I was still playing the judge. I thought I had come so far and dug so deep, how could that still be a judgment? Well, it was.

I looked at him, barely knowing what to say. "I don't understand" is all that came out.

He responded, "How about this. If you think they did the best they could, sit right here and tell me: How. Much. Better. Should. They. Have. Done?" He said that part louder and more slowly, one word at a time with staccato pauses in between, and suddenly it hit me. By saying that they did the best they could, I was literally saying that from my perspective, it would have been better for me if they had acted differently, if only they could have.

The root of the problem wasn't that I was saying it, it was that deep down, I believed it. I thought I had let go of everything, but instead I had practiced just enough acceptance to take the edge off the edgiest of my anger and find a gentler way to phrase it. To truly let go, I did two important things.

First, I got to the point where I could see that I was still suffering from the pains of judging them and holding onto resentment toward them. My judgment and resentment were my wrongs. Their behavior might have been wrong, too, but that is between them and God.

The second part took more time and more prayers, but to be free, I needed to offer them true unconditional forgiveness. This means moving past "they did the best they could" into "they did not know what they were doing." They. Did. Not. Know. Not in the sense of being consciously unaware of it mentally, but in a spiritual sense.

"Forgive them, they know not what they do," rather than "Forgive them because I have judged them as doing the best they could have done." It might take some time to get there or to even understand, but if you choose to take the time with it in prayer and meditation, you will get there, because I did, and if I did, you can, too.

In the meantime, I'll try my best to explain. They know not what they do means that they were running on their own past programming without realizing it. They were blind to their own behavior and its effects. No matter how much I want to argue that they knew, which, of course, I did argue at first, after enough prayer, I could see that they didn't know. They did not look at each other on their wedding day, pray together, and say, "Yes, after much contemplation and prayer, we have decided to make a family and then break it up and see what happens; let's see what happens to the kids in particular, you know, whether they end up confused and angry." It was not the plan.

Even for the situations for which I genuinely believed that someone was sinister enough that it *was* the plan, the point remains, and whoever is involved just came from a background with even more pain and confusion leading to even wackier programming, and to heal, I still had to pray until I could see that they did not know what they were doing.

Just to be crystal clear, this applies not only to parents but to anyone who I used to have judgment toward for their behavior. What about that "abusive ex"? Wasn't it enough for me to realize that he carried a lot of pain and was doing the best he could at the time? No, no, it was not, for that was a judgment of him, and one that was only hurting me. For me to totally heal, I had to pray until I could feel in my heart that he didn't know what he was doing. He was spiritually asleep. If he was spiritually awake, none of it would have happened. If I was spiritually awake enough to know the pain my past actions were going to cause others or the extent to which they would weigh on me, I wouldn't have done them either.

Today, I no longer determine whether anyone is doing the best they can or not. That's not up to me to figure out or judge. This is true for every happening, every hurt, every pain, every wound. By the power of God's grace moving into my heart through prayers for relief from my judgments and resentment, I can love—not judge, not even just accept, but love—every experience, even ones not shared here that might be viewed as traumatic, as a piece of my story, my path, and my growth.

It takes time, but for each situation, past and present, I pray until the reality that they did not know hits me like a ton of bricks. For the tough ones, it usually comes with tears of relief. Total forgiveness is always available. This isn't an easy one to process, but I promise it is one that is possible. And to be clear, the lesson here wasn't for me to change how I talk about my past, it was to dig deep enough that the way I talk about my past is changed.

Lesson 47

The Resentment Paradox

When my husband, Kevin, was young, his mom used to make sugar cookies. When she finished the dough, she would put it in the refrigerator and tell him and his siblings not to touch it. Kevin had trouble not touching it. He would sneak into the fridge and grab some dough to eat. But within a short time, he would begin to feel the remorse and regret associated with his guilt. When his mom called to him, he would hide. His mom was the last person he wanted to see. When the guilt escalated enough, he would even plot to run away from home. The guilt had taken over, and suddenly, his mind told him that home was awful. She was a bad mom. He needed to escape.

The conscience is a very finicky thing. Although in some ways it still baffles me to this day, I have come to understand that most often, the people I resent are not the people who have harmed me, but the people I have harmed. As a result of my guilt, I have created a chasm of dislike, distaste, or even hatred. In this example, Kevin stole from his mom, and within a short time, he had a resentment against her. She was what was keeping him from his beloved cookie dough, and he would have none of that. He stole the cookie dough, but now he was the one with resentment.

Moreover, resentment tends to escalate over time because we often experience consequences to our own harm. So, imagine if his mom had found out and then put him on a time-out, or perhaps told him he could not have cookies the rest of the day. He would resent her for this. But when it comes down to it, he is just resenting someone for their response to the harm he caused.

Allow me to share two other examples from my own life. The first occurred around 2015. I was at a house party at an Airbnb that my sister and her then husband had rented in my hometown over Christmas. She went to bed, and I ended up snorting her husband's medication off a countertop. I heard her coming down the stairs, and my best intoxicated cover-up was to cover the evidence with a trash can. The trash can on the counter was a tip-off to her that something was not right, and she removed it from the counter, revealing the lines of medication. She was furious. She yelled at me. I slept outside on the porch. The next day, she called my mom and told her what she'd witnessed, evidence that I had a drug problem. Now, I was furious and carrying a grudge. I did not want to see her. From my perspective, she was overreacting. I could not believe how rude she had been to me or that she had involved my mom. I carried a deep resentment for a long time. But the root of the resentment was not what she did, it was actually that I'd harmed her with what I did.

Let me try one last example. I cheated on every boyfriend I ever had up until I got sober, almost always during blackouts. Each time, without fail, I ended up resenting the boyfriend. I would proclaim, only upon being caught, of course, that I had realized that we had been growing apart, that he should have called me more, that he had been rude to me earlier that day, or the like. Unless his response was to take me back, I of course now had yet another reason to resent him. So, I then resented him not only for the reasons I had created to deny my guilt in my own conscience, but also because he wouldn't take me back. The real problem here is not what he did, it's that I cheated.

Of course, the dynamics of relationships are much more complicated, but it almost always goes back to the harm I did, even if my harm is something like incessant nagging, trying to control another person, or confusing others with erratic behavior. The root is still the harm done by my actions.

I'll end with a metaphor that came to me the other day. I was riding as a passenger in a sidecar motorcycle that Kevin was driving. I suddenly felt a pain in my arm, then another. I realized that a wasp had flown into the sleeve of my jacket. It was trapped and left with no choice but to sting me. In this metaphor, my sleeve is me and the wasp is those I resent. I knowingly or unknowingly harm others, and I often do not even realize I am harming them. I just realize that they are stinging me. Then all I see is that I resent them for stinging me, when the real work is understanding how I am behaving like the sleeve.

It is only by sitting down in self-examination that I realize that I am the sleeve, putting others in situations in which they have no choice but to behave in self-protective ways that I perceive as harmful and then resent. But there would be no sting if I had not trapped them in my sleeve. And so it is with life; most people I resent are people that I harmed, who never otherwise would have behaved in ways that I perceived as harmful to me.

Having resentments against lots of people is not an indicator that lots of people have harmed me, it's an indicator that *I have harmed a lot of people*. It isn't until I realize this that I am on a path to reparation—and on a path on which I can hopefully catch myself before I accidentally or purposefully become a sleeve.

Lesson 48

How to Let Go of Resentment

For the first twenty-nine years of my life, I was unaware that I was chock-full of resentment. The gift and the curse of soothers like alcohol and drugs is that they allow one to keep living in the delusion that all is well. At age twenty-nine, with alcohol and drugs removed from my life, it became abundantly clear to me that I was uncomfortable in my own skin and that the nature of much of that discomfort was suppressed resentment. Furthermore, I had come to understand that holding on to those resentments was only harming me—that resentment was like drinking poison and expecting someone else to feel the harmful effects. So, I wanted to be free from resentment, but I did not know how to go about doing that.

The first step toward freedom from resentment was coming to understand that there are two distinct pieces to the pain of resentment: the pain of my unforgiveness and the pain of my anger. The next step was to realize that to heal these, I was going to need God's help. That is because one highly important piece of the puzzle is that making the decision to no longer want to resent someone is not the same as doing so. The former is an intellectual task, the latter is a spiritual task. Wanting to forgive someone and wanting to let go of my anger toward them are intellectual tasks, doing so is a spiritual task.

Saying "I have forgiven them" is not the same as forgiving them. It is a lot like people who have made an intellectual decision to believe in God, but then do not actually pray to God nor let God guide their decision-making. Sure, they believe in God intellectually, but it will not actually change their life until they carry out that decision spiritually. Similarly, I must actually do spiritual work to let go of resentment. I cannot just decide that I am not angry anymore.

Hopefully, I have convinced you of the importance of the spiritual work of letting go of resentment beyond the intellectual decision to no longer resent. But just what does that entail? For me, this is what it looks like. First, I get very clear on exactly what I am angry about. If I can't see it, I ask for God's help. I then identify exactly how this has affected me. Is it my financial security, my personal security, my self-esteem, my ambitions, or something else that has been harmed? It is important to realize that resentment is really all about me. We do not resent others unless whatever they have done affects us.

Next, I pray, not just once, but repeatedly, until I feel some type of shift. The shift is different for every resentment, but I wait until I feel a physical, emotional, or mental shift of some kind. Sometimes I burp, sometimes a montage of past situations plays through my mind as I let go of each one, sometimes I feel peace, and sometimes my mind goes blank and I forget what I was just praying about. But just trust yourself and wait for the shift. Sometimes it happens after a few prayers, sometimes it takes days or weeks and hundreds of prayers, but it always comes eventually.

This is the prayer that I use. "God *help me* show ____ the same tolerance, pity, and patience I would cheerfully grant a sick friend. They are spiritually sick. How can I help them? God *save me* from being angry. Thy will be done." I have italicized the two most important pieces of this prayer, which clearly show that I am not so much praying for the other person as I am praying for myself.

With this prayer, I am asking God to help me show them the same tolerance, pity, and patience that I would cheerfully grant a sick friend. In other words, I am asking God for help forgiving them. Second, I am asking for God to save me from my anger toward them, in other words, to forgive me for my anger. The middle of the prayer is basically just a blessing upon whomever I am angry at. And it ends with a prayer for God's will. But the important pieces are God helping me forgive them and God saving me from being angry at them, because what I really need is salvation from my own mistakes, and those mistakes are anger and unforgiveness.

So, in short, any time I identify that I have moved or am moving toward resentment, I repeat this prayer again and again, and every time, I eventually feel a shift. Some shifts are more dramatic than others, but a shift always comes.

With the shift comes the final letting go of the resentment, which is when I realize that none of the effects were ever the other person's fault. It was the pain of my anger and unforgiveness that I was feeling. I know this to be true because every time I use this prayer, the anger and unforgiveness are gone, and with that, I am no longer in pain. And yet, nothing else has changed. The past is still the past. Whatever happened still happened. But God very much changes my reaction to it. And what a beautiful experience it is to realize that all the pain comes from within, and that all peace comes from God. The only thing that lies in between resentment and peace is the spiritual work of letting go.

Lesson 49

Stop Trying to Rationalize and Justify Others' Behavior

The other day, while driving down the road...well, nothing happened that I am aware of, and that's the most interesting fact of all. Let me explain. As far as I can remember, not a single person sped past me, cut me off, pulled off in the wrong place, spent too long at a red light, drove too slowly in front of me, drove too slowly in the wrong lane, did not use their blinker, or used their blinker too soon or too late. That was also true the day before and last week as well. Was it because Minnesota drivers were having the best driving month ever? No, it was not. By the end of the essay, you'll know the reason.

But first, let's go back to a day in the life of Lisa a few years ago. I call this living in my lower nature; I was just reacting to life—spirituality level zero. My day was filled with frustration about how other people were behaving, both on and off the road. But here, I am going to stick to examples on the road. People were driving the wrong way, according to me, and I was being affected. I was frustrated. I wished that they weren't driving the way that they were. I noticed it, and it was, at best, annoying, and most of the time it was infuriating. I stayed frustrated until I could vent to someone, grab a drink, exercise, or do whatever else I could do to blow off steam that day—never asking myself why I was full of steam.

Now, here's a day in the life of Lisa beginning her journey in spirituality but mostly caught in psychology rather than spirituality. The scene: A car went flying past me. I would begin to react, but then I would instead try to calm my anger by rationalizing and justifying their behavior. Perhaps she is pregnant and on the way to the hospital. Perhaps they are late for work and will lose their job if they are late one more time. Perhaps they must drop off a highly important document somewhere before closing time. I would tell myself that I did not know their story, and that if I did, I might understand their behavior. This implied that there were also possible stories for which I would not give them a pass on their behavior.

However, even if I did give them a pass, rationalizing and justifying their behavior was unknowingly sinking me deeper into despair, often a consequence of well-intentioned psychological tools. What do I mean by this? At the moment that I tried to justify their behavior, I was ignoring my own wrong; namely, the anger that I had just built toward this stranger and my judgment of their behavior. Instead of recognizing my wrong and doing something about it, I was using tactics that suppressed my anger toward them while denying my guilt about judging them, which was a recipe for sinking deeper into despair in the long run.

In the case of someone else's driving, one might argue that the wrong I'd just committed in judging the other driver was a rather minor moral infraction, and they would be right. But I have found that what I do in small and perhaps less important situations is generally indicative of what I would do in larger, more important situations with greater consequences.

So, the question is, what do I do now in circumstances great and small, and how is that related to the fact that drivers in Minnesota all appear to have recently attended driving school? Whenever I catch myself trying to suppress my own anger through rationalization and justification, I instead recognize that at that very moment, I am making a judgment against another person, and I turn to prayer. I ask God to save me from my own anger and judgment toward this person and direct my attention to His will for me instead. In other words, I confess my wrong.

What has been profound to experience is the compounding effect of using justification and rationalization over and over again compared to the compounding effect of using prayer over and over again. The compounding effect of my old approach was that I continued to notice and judge others' behavior and would, therefore, have to continue to come up with more and more excuses for such behaviors. However, the compounding effect of prayer is that slowly but surely, I notice less and less of other people's behavior.

I know it sounds impossible, but it's not only my experience with drivers on the road, it's my experience with every behavior. The more that I can catch myself judging and confess my wrong, the less I judge. Judgment begets more judgment, anger begets more anger, but confession of my wrong begets more and more peace.

Trying to justify and rationalize another person's behavior is simply choosing the circumstances under which I am willing to justify my own judgment of them. Confession of my wrong in judging them gets me to a place where I can love them regardless of their behavior and eventually, more often than otherwise, not notice their behavior at all.

Lesson 50

My Pain Is Not Their Fault

In high school, I was an accomplished runner; honestly, this was in part—or perhaps almost entirely—because of an exercise compulsion related to an eating disorder along with the approval and validation I received from winning races. But I digress. This story is about a particular ten-mile trail race. About a half mile into the race, I tripped on a root and tumbled down a hill. I could feel that there was blood running down my shin, but I didn't want to look. I just kept running. I made it to the finish line 9.5 miles later with a gaping wound on my shin that then needed stitches. It had split further and further open throughout the race, and by the end, it was full of dirt and dust, ripe for infection. I did get the wound cleaned and stitched up that day. So, although I didn't deal with the wound the moment it happened, it wasn't long before I started making moves toward healing. Today, it is healed, the whole experience rarely comes to mind, and my leg is in no pain. However, had I not dealt with it that day, had I just let it sit open for the next fifteen years, I would have an infected, painful mess on my hands right now. References to running might even be triggering.

This is not meant to be a lesson on physical pain and healing, rather it is a metaphor for spiritual pain and healing. Imagine if I had just gone on telling everyone about all the pain I was in while doing nothing about the wound because I was the victim. "Oh, you want to tell me there is something I can do? I don't want to listen to you. You don't understand." With a gaping physical wound, most people would suggest I take steps toward healing. But when the pain is spiritual, people not only let me spread infection all over myself and others, but they also validate me for doing so. "You're so strong, and he was abusive." "You're right, she was awful to you." "What you did is nothing in comparison to what they did." No one ever told me to begin the healing process by examining myself. Instead, I went around blaming others' actions for my spiritual pain when my current pain wasn't their fault for two reasons.

The first reason is that most of the time, I caused the pain. In the case of this running metaphor, although my inclination is to blame the root for my pain, the real problem was that I wasn't paying attention to my footing, and so I tripped on the root. I can blame the root. But ultimately, it is my fault for not paying attention. If I go back further, I wanted approval for being in a long and challenging race. Moreover, there's a good chance I was up late with friends the night before, and perhaps I was drinking; and most likely, given my eating disorder, I hadn't eaten breakfast. My judgment was totally compromised by my own actions. I quickly began to see that although it first appeared that the root was my problem, my trouble was of my own making—I had literally caused it.

This example is about a root and a physical wound, but the same principle applies to spiritual pain and blaming others for hurting me. More often than not, I did something to cause the situation that led them to harm me. I drank too much, I nagged, I tried to control a situation, I escalated a fight, I lied, I cheated, I wanted that guy to flirt with me and then it went too far, and the list goes on. In other words, I was selfish and so were they, but I then chose to only look at how they were to blame rather than how I was to blame.

I used to say that I had an abusive ex. I now say that I was in a relationship where there was a lot of confusion because I see how my actions contributed to the escalation of our altercations. I blamed my ex in the same way that I blamed the root. It doesn't mean he wasn't wrong, that's between him and God, but I had not taken the time to understand my own faults and clean those up with God.

The second reason my pain is not their fault is that whether I contributed to the occurrence of harm or not, if I am still in pain today, it is because I am choosing to not go to God to let go of it. I am no longer suffering the pain of the harm; I am suffering from the pain of holding onto it. Let's change the running metaphor to fit the most extreme version of this scenario. This time, someone has placed the root in my way with the intent to trip me. Let's say this was a malicious person with whom I had no previous interaction and that their doing this was zero percent my fault.

If I am still suffering from the pain of the wound fifteen years later because I chose never to clean it or get stitches, is that the fault of the malicious person or is that my fault? Of course, it is my fault. I am not in pain because of what they did, I am in pain because I never dealt with it, be it minor harm or a major trauma. If I am still suffering years later because of the harm done to me, if I still get anxiety every time I look at the scar or am triggered by people running, I am not suffering from their actions but from the pain of my resentment and unforgiveness—period.

The reality is that we all suffer from acute reactions. We get angry, we get hurt, we feel abandoned, we feel betrayed, we feel embarrassed. However, when those feelings last for more than a short time, the other person is no longer to blame. I am to blame. I can choose to turn to God to deal with the pain as quickly as it builds up. Or I can choose to sit in blame, anger, and unforgiveness, and let my anxiety and sensitivity build up. The choice is mine. But I better not blame the pain of anger and unforgiveness on the other person. That one is all on me.

How do I know? Because I used to live in constant pain, anxiety, and despair, and by turning my anger and unforgiveness over to God, today I do not have these feelings. As long as I remained unwilling to go to God to let go of my anger and unforgiveness, I remained in pain. As soon as I became willing to turn to God with all of it, the pain fell away. I have sat across from many women who have become willing to do the same, and they have found the same relief.

So, my pain is my fault because about 90 percent of the time, if I really search my soul, by my own choices and actions, I have caused the harm to occur and haven't gone to God with my faults, and 100 percent of the time, I am at fault for not turning to God to let go of my lingering anger and unforgiveness. This is not bad news, though, nor a reason to sit in self-pity, because as soon as I accept this, the good news is that I can turn to God, and, in prayer, admit the wrong of my own choices and actions, the wrong of my anger and unforgiveness, or perhaps both, and then the relief of God's grace comes and the pain is over. There is no timeline. God lets me decide when I am ready to let go of the pain, and He is always ready and waiting.

Lesson 51

Stop Asking People for Forgiveness

I got married last summer, and as part of preparation for that marriage, my then fiancé and I attended an engaged couples retreat. Many of the lectures given at the retreat were useful, especially for couples who may have trouble communicating about important issues such as finances or extended family expectations. However, one lecture caught me very off guard, especially since the retreat was billed as spiritual in nature.

The lecture was about asking your partner for forgiveness. The assignment was to make a list of things for which you want to ask your partner's forgiveness, read it to them, and then ask for forgiveness. I would have stopped in my tracks, but I was already sitting. Not only was this the assignment for the weekend, but this was also described as the foundation of how we should act in a relationship. I must have signed up for the wrong retreat; this was supposed to be spiritual marriage preparation, not codependency training.

Don't get me wrong. There was a time in my life when I would have been totally on board with this. When I had no relationship with God, there was really no choice but to seek forgiveness from other people, making me totally dependent on them. But this was a retreat that was supposedly God-centered. Suddenly, it was very human-centered, perhaps even codependency-centered.

If my being forgiven depends on getting forgiveness from you...if my being at peace depends on you deciding to forgive me...if I think my soul can be healed by other humans, I am in deep trouble.

Let me clarify with an example. In previous relationships, I had cheated on my partner. I would come back and cry, tell them I was sorry, and ask them to forgive me. It would sound something like, "Baby, I'm sorry, please forgive me." In return, after some crying or arguing, they often said something like, "Babe, I love you and I know you're sorry, I forgive you." We would both get a hit of dopamine for reuniting and think we had put it behind us. That was all fine and dandy until the next blow-up fight or the next time someone cheated. Most likely, this was happening because I didn't see my behavior as inherently wrong nor get to the bottom of what was causing me to cheat. I didn't wake up to the reality of my behavior. I just got him to forgive me.

No real forgiveness happened because the problem was never whether I could get my partner to forgive me, it was whether I could truly understand in my heart that my behavior was wrong and bring that to God for forgiveness.

I was wrong. I was trapped in lust. I was blinded by the need for male approval. I was selfish and self-absorbed. I was dishonest. My partner did not have the ability to forgive nor heal those things. Only God can do that. It was certainly healthy for them to forgive me, whether they broke up with me or not. What isn't healthy is that I was seeking forgiveness from my partner rather than from God. In fact, if I went to a spiritually healthy person and asked them for forgiveness, they should tell me to take my sorrows to God.

In my marriage today, I occasionally make mistakes or commit acts of wrongdoing that hurt my husband, and he occasionally does the same to me. We both take our wrongdoing directly to God. It is only then that I go to Kevin and tell him that I was wrong for whatever I did. You will never catch us seeking forgiveness from one another. I repeat, asking for forgiveness from him is not something I do, it simply makes no sense and solves no problems except for giving me the perception, true or false, that he is no longer angry. In other words, it is not at all effective in healing my soul, it is only effective in giving me a little hit of the neurotransmitter dopamine. That's not healing, that's just codependency.

It is also quite manipulative. Think of it this way; you are essentially saying, "I know I hurt you, but now I have one more favor to ask. I would really like to feel better, and my feelings are totally dependent on whether I get approval from you or not. If you could forgive me so that I can sleep well knowing that you approve of me again, that would be amazing." I know I would never use those words, but it doesn't make my intention any less codependent.

Letting my peace depend on other humans isn't intimacy. There was no spiritual development as long as I was leaning on other humans for forgiveness. But when I started taking that wrongdoing to God for forgiveness, I not only saw my spiritual development vastly improve, but also my ability to have true intimacy with others.

Lesson 52

What Will Your Gravestone Say?

I wish I had not cheated on him. I wish I would have been nicer that time. Can you imagine if that shot in the soccer game had been just two inches over to the left? That goal would have changed my life. What if I had won that award? What if I hadn't dropped out of that class? What if he hadn't treated me that way? What if I had just held my tongue? I wish I never even brought that up. If only I would have made it to that party. If only I had applied to that college. If I had different parents, my life would be different. If I had grown up in a different town, my life would be different. Imagine if I had just found a way to get along with my siblings. If I had never met that guy, I would never have tried drugs. If I didn't drink that one day, I wouldn't be in this position. If she hadn't said that to me, I wouldn't be the way I am.

Sound familiar? That is the internal dialogue of a person with a gravestone that would read, "I wish it would have been different." I used to live my life partially in my life and partially in various delusions about how it could have been different or how it might be different in the future. I wasn't really living. I wasn't enjoying my life. I was just trying to work out why I didn't get what I thought I wanted on the timeline that I thought I wanted it. That's not living, that is just trying not to die.

Have you ever thought about what might be on your gravestone? Or perhaps a better way to state it is, "How are you living your life?" Do you wish it would have been different? Is that what you spend your time thinking about?

Today, I am inching toward a gravestone that simply reads, "That sure was fun!" There's no reminiscing about how my life could have or should have been different; no attachment to whether it becomes different in the future, just living.

How does that happen? What is the difference between a person living their life in a state of "I wish it would have been different," and one living in a state of "That sure was fun!"? The answer is forgiveness.

I have come to realize that the only difference between being able to wear life as a loose garment, take it as it comes, and live life on life's terms is how quickly and thoroughly I can identify and resolve resentment. Every single one of the statements at the beginning of this essay can be boiled down to some type of resentment, because if everyone had done exactly what I wanted or expected them to do, my life would have had no regrets. If X had not happened, Y would not have happened. If X had not happened, I would not have done Y. Every time, if I look far enough back, someone did something that I wished they had not done, and then I held onto it.

The resentment might be in the form of jealousy, envy, frustration, or fear, but it's always there. I know that because when my conscience is clear of resentments (that I am aware of), I can look at my life and not wish that a single thing was different. When I start wishing something was different, I know it is time to pause and figure out what resentment I am harboring.

Sometimes that can sound callous. For example, is it fair to the people I lied to or cheated on to say that I do not wish a single thing was different? Absolutely. I often remind people that just because someone else does not have the capacity to forgive does not mean that you need to hold yourself in condemnation. If you have truly healed from it, you will not repeat it, and you can help others out of the trap that they are in. If you had not done it, you could not be helpful now.

So today, life sure is fun. I do not regret the past nor wish to pretend that it did not happen. It all happened. I do not wish that any of it was different. I watch God use my story to heal others every single day if I am willing to let Him, and that sure is fun! So, perhaps it's time to ask yourself—is your gravestone going to say "I wish it would have been different" or "That sure was fun"?

Afterword

If you made it this far, I applaud you, especially if you read all fifty-two lessons and didn't just skip straight to the end to see what was here. If you did skip to the end, I get it. I have done that same thing. Now go back and start from the beginning, and I promise you'll thank me later.

Assuming you read the book to here, you have read through lessons that may have stirred up a lot for you. I know this might feel like a bad thing, but I promise it's a good thing. Imagine a jar full of dirt and water. For years, you were likely sitting there thinking that you were clear, but it was just because all the dirt had sunk to the bottom. While reading this book, you may have stirred up the dirt and cleared some of it out. Or you might be sitting here reading this feeling as though you are now a jar of mud. Trust me, I know the feeling. Stay in prayer, even if you don't quite believe in God yet. The more you pray, the faster the filtration.

The greatest gift of awakening is clarity—clarity of perception and accuracy of response in every situation. I don't bring my past into the present, nor do I drag my future into the present. At any given moment, I have cleared all the dirt I am aware of, and, therefore, I can live and react to life sanely and normally. And if I ever get a little off-kilter, I know I have just accidentally let a little dirt in or perhaps stirred some up that was previously stuck, and I turn right to the God I used to not believe in to clear it up.

I promise, one day at a time, it gets better and better. Now, maybe start the book over, and as you read each lesson again, you'll realize how far you've come.

Finally, the reason I write is in the hope that one more person gets it, that one more person heals, that one more person wakes up and sees life differently. If that's you, please reach out and let me know. I read every message I get, and I would love nothing more than for the next one to be from you.

Thank you. I love you, truly. Not as much as God does, but I love you as much as I am able given where I am today with my spiritual growth. And that's quite a bit.

—**Lisa**

Acknowledgements

I want to start by acknowledging my mother, Carol, as she has read and edited almost every word I have ever written. She also has unendingly supported all my ideas and projects, even when she can't see how they are going to end up. Her chosen path has always been unwavering support of me no matter my endeavor. I want to acknowledge my father, because long talks with him over the years about the meaning of human existence have been important to my developing a curiosity for the deeper questions in life. I also want to acknowledge my stepparents and all my siblings for always being there for me, even when they were baffled by my life choices.

I want to acknowledge my best friend, Brooklyn. I met her and my husband at the same Christmas morning recovery meeting in 2020. My life was not only changed by meeting him, but also by meeting her. It has been an honor and a joy to walk every step of my spiritual path with her, through laughter and through tears. She is the kind of friend who always points me back to God and is not afraid to unabashedly cheer me on or call me out, depending on what I need. And she somehow always knows what I need. I want to acknowledge all the other men and women who have supported me on this path over the last few years: Caroline, Michele, Breanna, Dave, Peter, Mariana, Aunt Jean, Alexa, Claire, Sue, Hailey, Alex, Michaela, Sherry, Julie, Kristine, Paul, Amanda, Kira, Emma, Jane, Father Jacob, Maggie, and many others. I want to thank all the members of the Solutions on Second Street and Mixed Hazelnuts recovery meetings. Without you, I most likely wouldn't even be alive.

I want to acknowledge the women of my Monday night small group. Without the class on spiritual gifts that we all took together, I never would have even considered writing about my spiritual journey. I want to acknowledge the women in my 2023–2024 BSF Tuesday morning group and my St. Olaf Wednesday night group for your unending prayers of support.

I want to acknowledge my dear friend, Karen Casey. Her belief in me as a writer and her support throughout the writing of this book has meant the world to me.

I want to acknowledge Brenda, my acquiring editor and the publisher of Mango, not only for her guidance and support through the publishing process, but also for taking a chance on me.

I want to acknowledge my high school friends from the graduating class of 2009 of Lancaster Country Day School—some of my most preeminent supporters and cheerleaders.

I want to acknowledge all my friends and mentors from my college and graduate school years who have come back into my life over these last few years of sobriety and those among them who have always been there to support me and to tell me to go get help when I needed it, especially Alex, Molly, Dana, Mary, Brittany, Emily, and Dylan.

I want to acknowledge the early supporters of my original Instagram account, The Sober Essayist. Without your likes and shares, my writing would have never made it anywhere other than into the hands of my own friends and family. I also want to acknowledge every person who follows, likes, comments on, and shares my content today on @drlisastanton. It truly means the world to have a community of people who want to share and spread God-centered spiritual growth online.

I want to acknowledge my husband, Kevin. Without him, this book would not be possible because he is not only my partner in life, but also one of my greatest spiritual teachers.

The list of others who have had a profound impact on me and on this book is long, but for now, I thank you all, those listed here and those not listed. And of course, I thank the one and only God, Creator of all good things, including this book.

About the Author

Never in a million years did Lisa Stanton think she would be writing a book like this. Her scientific roots were deep, but her awakening over the last few years has been strong. Lisa holds a bachelor's degree in psychology from the University of Richmond and a PhD in social psychology from the University of Minnesota. Her expertise is in behavior change theory and applications. During graduate school, she was named the student advisory council chair for the Society for Health Psychology, a division of the American Psychological Association, and was a finalist for a National Science Foundation Graduate Research Fellowship. After finishing her PhD, she spent two years in the Department of Preventive Medicine at Northwestern Feinberg School of Medicine in Chicago, Illinois, where she completed a National Cancer Institute T32 postdoctoral research fellowship in Behavioral Cancer Prevention and Control. During graduate school and her postdoctoral fellowship, she taught or assisted in the teaching of eighteen undergraduate and master's level courses. She has co-authored thirty academic publications and several encyclopedia entries and book chapters. She has spoken at numerous psychology conferences across the United States and in Europe. Before starting her most recent writing endeavors, she worked remotely for a year and a half as a researcher for a health technology start-up in Mountain View, California.

Despite her vast educational background, you will find neither psychology nor behavior change theory in the solutions offered in the pages of *52 Life-Changing Lesson I Learned in Recovery*. Her recent writings are about her personal experiences in recovery from not only addiction, but also eating disorders, anxiety conditions, ADHD, IBS, alopecia areata, and more. She writes about her journey from the belief that more scientific knowledge would solve all her problems to her experience that a relationship with God does so. These writings appear on her Instagram page @drlisastanton, which is enjoyed by thousands of followers. Lisa currently lives in Minnesota with her husband. They share a love of service and spend their days helping others who are suffering, whether from addiction or eating disorders, or just a person in need. Their favorite activities include sharing meals with friends and family, motorcycling both on their own bikes and together on their sidecar motorcycle, making year-round visits to ice-cream shops for dessert, and traveling—especially on cruises with silent discos and to see their many friends and family around the country and the world.

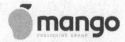

Mango Publishing, established in 2014, publishes an eclectic list of books by diverse authors—both new and established voices—on topics ranging from business, personal growth, women's empowerment, LGBTQ studies, health, and spirituality to history, popular culture, time management, decluttering, lifestyle, mental wellness, aging, and sustainable living. We were named 2019 *and* 2020's #1 fastest growing independent publisher by *Publishers Weekly*. Our success is driven by our main goal, which is to publish high-quality books that will entertain readers as well as make a positive difference in their lives.

Our readers are our most important resource; we value your input, suggestions, and ideas. We'd love to hear from you—after all, we are publishing books for you!

Please stay in touch with us and follow us at:

Facebook: Mango Publishing
Twitter: @MangoPublishing
Instagram: @MangoPublishing
LinkedIn: Mango Publishing
Pinterest: Mango Publishing
Newsletter: mangopublishinggroup.com/newsletter

Join us on Mango's journey to reinvent publishing, one book at a time.

www.ingramcontent.com/pod-product-compliance
Lightning Source LLC
Jackson TN
JSHW032156050425
82084JS00005B/5

* 9 7 8 1 6 8 4 8 1 7 0 5 4 *